THE VISUAL
DICTIONARY *of the*
SKELETON

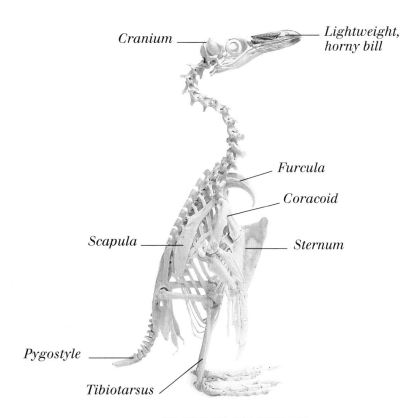

Cranium

Lightweight, horny bill

Furcula

Coracoid

Scapula

Sternum

Pygostyle

Tibiotarsus

PENGUIN SKELETON

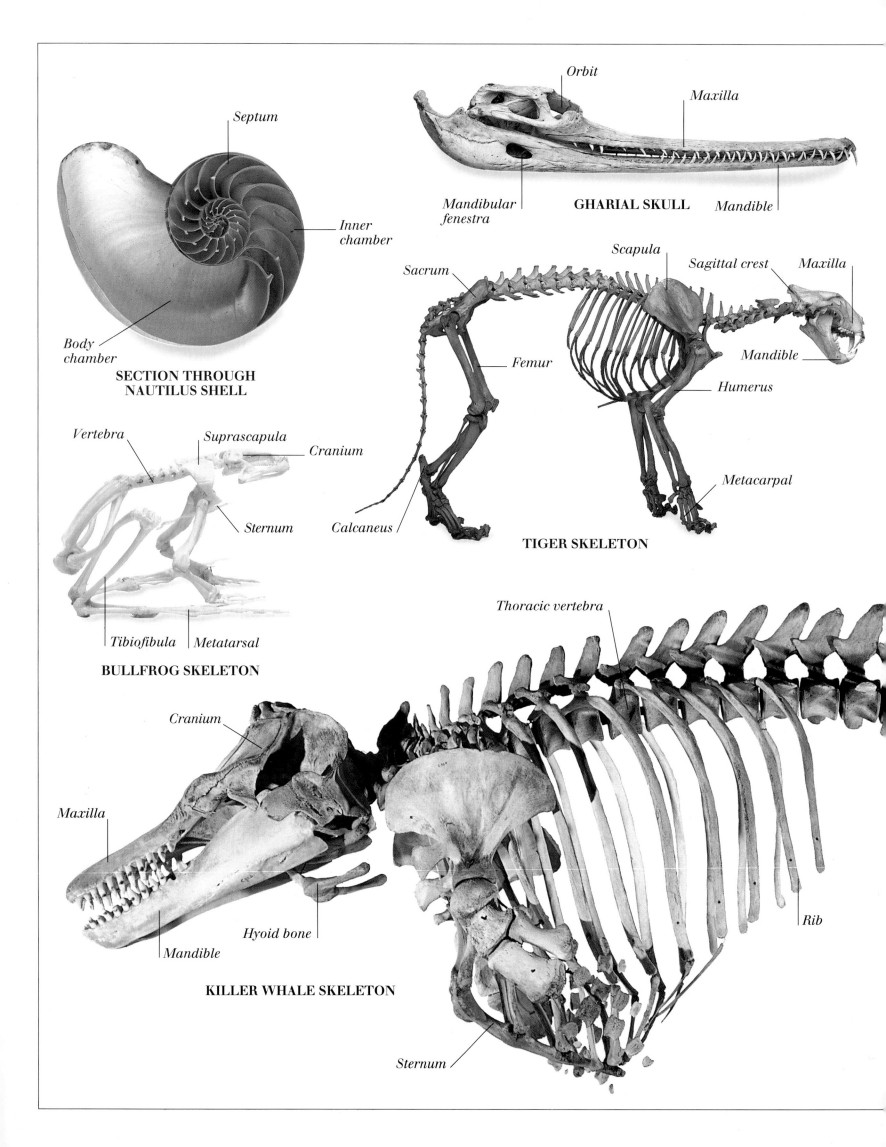

Septum

SECTION THROUGH NAUTILUS SHELL

Inner chamber

Body chamber

Orbit

Maxilla

GHARIAL SKULL

Mandibular fenestra

Mandible

Sacrum

Scapula

Sagittal crest

Maxilla

Femur

Mandible

Humerus

Metacarpal

Calcaneus

TIGER SKELETON

Vertebra

Suprascapula

Cranium

Sternum

Tibiofibula

Metatarsal

BULLFROG SKELETON

Thoracic vertebra

Cranium

Maxilla

Rib

Hyoid bone

Mandible

Sternum

KILLER WHALE SKELETON

THE VISUAL
DICTIONARY *of the*
SKELETON

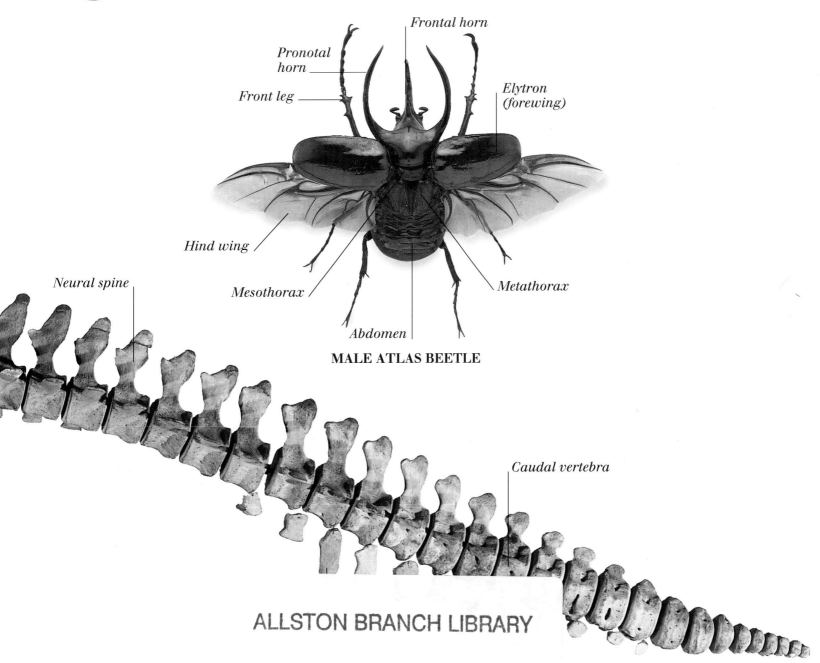

Frontal horn

Pronotal horn

Front leg

Elytron (forewing)

Hind wing

Neural spine

Mesothorax

Metathorax

Abdomen

MALE ATLAS BEETLE

Caudal vertebra

DK PUBLISHING, INC

A DK PUBLISHING BOOK

PROJECT ART EDITOR CHRIS WALKER
DESIGNER HELEN BENFIELD

PROJECT EDITOR FIONA COURTENAY-THOMPSON
EDITORIAL ASSISTANT WILL HODGKINSON
CONSULTANT EDITOR DR. RICHARD WALKER

US EDITOR JILL HAMILTON
US CONSULTANT JAYMIE L. BRAUER, AMERICAN MUSEUM OF NATURAL HISTORY

MANAGING ART EDITOR BRYN WALLS
MANAGING EDITORS RUTH MIDGLEY, MARTYN PAGE

ILLUSTRATIONS JOANNA CAMERON, DEBORAH MAIZELS, GRAHAM ROSEWARNE, JOHN TEMPERTON

PICTURE RESEARCH INGRID NILSSON

PRODUCTION HILARY STEPHENS

Caudal vertebra   *Thoracic vertebra*   *Scapula*   *Cranium*   *Maxilla*

Mandible

Metatarsal

MONITOR LIZARD SKELETON

FIRST AMERICAN EDITION, 1995

2 4 6 8 10 9 7 5 3
PUBLISHED IN THE UNITED STATES BY DK PUBLISHING, INC.,
95 MADISON AVENUE, NEW YORK, NEW YORK, 10016

COPYRIGHT © 1995
DORLING KINDERSLEY LIMITED, LONDON

DISTRIBUTED BY HOUGHTON MIFFLIN COMPANY, BOSTON.
VISIT US ON THE WORLD WIDE WEB AT
HTTP://WWW.DK.COM
LIBRARY OF CONGRESS CATALOGING-IN-PUBLICATION DATA
WALKER. RICHARD. 1951-
THE VISUAL DICTIONARY OF THE SKELETON / WRITTEN BY RICHARD WALKER.
— 1ST AMERICAN ED.
P.   CM. — (EYEWITNESS VISUAL DICTIONARIES)
INCLUDES INDEX.
ISBN 0-7894-0135-5
1. SKELETON—TERMINOLOGY—JUVENILE LITERATURE. 2. SKELETON—PICTORIAL WORKS—JUVENILE LITERATURE.
3. BONES—TERMINOLGY—JUVENILE LITERATURE. 4. BONES—PICTORIAL WORKS—JUVENILE LITERATURE.
5. PICTURE DICTIONARIES, ENGLISH—JUVENILE LITERATURE.
[1. SKELETON. 2. BONES 3. ANATOMY, COMPARATIVE.] I. TITLE. II. SERIES.
QL821.W17 1995
591.4'71—DC20   95-11956
                                CIP
                                AC

REPRODUCED BY COLOURSCAN, SINGAPORE
PRINTED AND BOUND BY ARNOLDO MONDADORI IN VERONA, ITALY

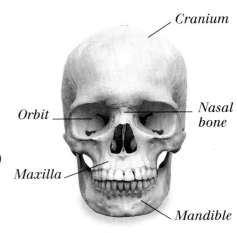

Prominent supraorbital ridge

Sloping forehead

Orbit

Deep, flat cheekbone

HOMO ERECTUS SKULL

Cranium

Orbit

Nasal bone

Maxilla

Mandible

HUMAN SKULL

Contents

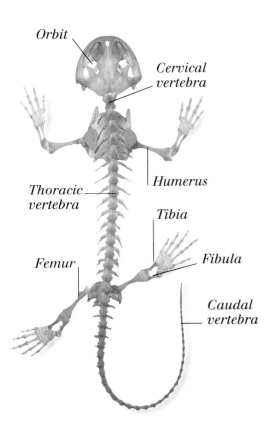

Skull

Coracoid

Cervical vertebra

Carapace

Marginal scute

Caudal vertebra

Femur

TURTLE SKELETON

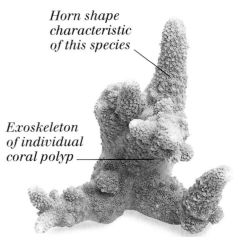

Horn shape characteristic of this species

Exoskeleton of individual coral polyp

CORAL COLONY SKELETON

Orbit

Cervical vertebra

Thoracic vertebra

Humerus

Tibia

Femur

Fibula

Caudal vertebra

SALAMANDER SKELETON

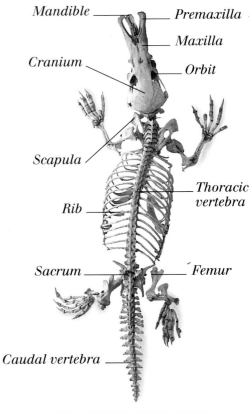

Mandible

Premaxilla

Maxilla

Cranium

Orbit

Scapula

Thoracic vertebra

Rib

Sacrum

Femur

Caudal vertebra

PLATYPUS SKELETON

Skeleton varieties 1

THE SKELETON IS A SUPPORTIVE framework that maintains the shape of an organism and protects its internal organs. In many animals, the skeleton also plays a vital role in movement. There are two main types of skeleton: internal skeletons (endoskeletons) and external skeletons (exoskeletons). Vertebrates (animals with backbones)—fish, amphibians, reptiles, birds, and mammals—have endoskeletons, which are usually made of bone. A few vertebrates, such as boxfish and tortoises, have both endoskeletons and exoskeletons. Most invertebrates (animals without backbones) have exoskeletons. These include the body cases of insects and crustaceans, the shells of snails, and the tests of sea urchins. Some single-celled organisms also have exoskeletons, for example the outer coat of diatoms. Other types of skeleton include the hydrostatic (fluid-filled) skeleton of earthworms, and plant skeletons, which are composed of various elements, such as xylem, that help support roots, stems, and leaves.

PARROT SKELETON

Orbit
Upper mandible
Cranium
Auditory meatus
Cervical vertebra
Bill
Humerus
Femur
Radius
Ulna
Pygostyle
Lower mandible
Pelvis
Metacarpal
Coracoid
Furcula
Digit
Sternum
Rib
Keel of sternum
Tibiotarsus
Claw
Phalanx
Tarsometatarsus

FROG SKELETON

Suprascapula
Cranium
Frontoparietal bone
Lumbar vertebra
Nasal bone
Sacral vertebra
Maxilla
Mandible
Scapula
Sternum
Femur
Humerus
Pelvis
Radio-ulna
Carpal
Tibiofibula
Metacarpal
Calcaneus
Astragalus
Metatarsal
Phalanx

LIZARD SKELETON

Metacarpal
Cranium
Phalanx
Orbit
Cervical vertebra
Carpal
Radius
Scapula
Ulna
Rib
Thoracolumbar vertebra
Sacrum
Femur
Pelvis
Tibia
Tarsal
Phalanx
Metatarsal
Caudal vertebra

CARP SKELETON

Dorsal fin
Parietal bone
Neural spine
Vertebra
Frontal bone
Orbit
Caudal fin
Dentary bone
Hemal spine
Rib
Pectoral fin
Maxilla
Anal fin
Interhemal
Pelvic fin
Opercular bone

BADGER SKELETON

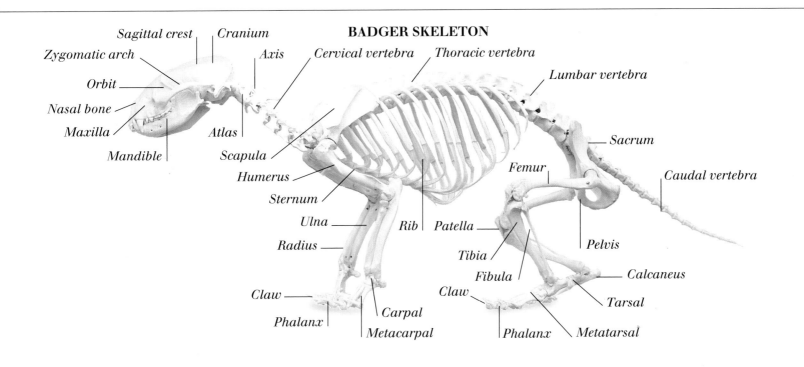

Sagittal crest
Zygomatic arch
Cranium
Axis
Cervical vertebra
Thoracic vertebra
Lumbar vertebra
Orbit
Nasal bone
Maxilla
Atlas
Sacrum
Mandible
Scapula
Femur
Humerus
Caudal vertebra
Sternum
Ulna
Rib
Patella
Pelvis
Radius
Tibia
Fibula
Calcaneus
Claw
Claw
Tarsal
Phalanx
Carpal
Phalanx
Metatarsal
Metacarpal

HUMAN SKELETON

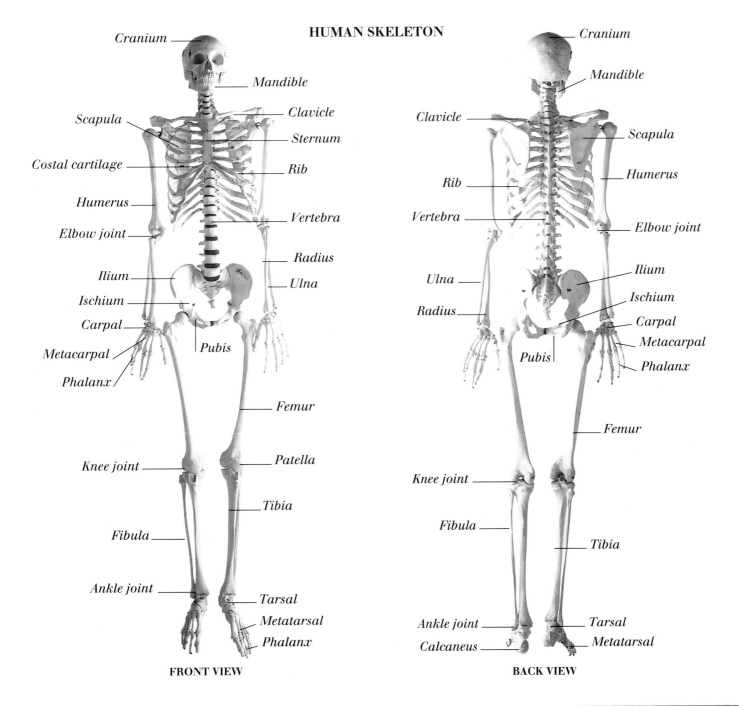

Cranium
Cranium
Mandible
Mandible
Clavicle
Scapula
Clavicle
Sternum
Scapula
Costal cartilage
Rib
Humerus
Rib
Humerus
Vertebra
Vertebra
Elbow joint
Elbow joint
Radius
Ilium
Ulna
Ilium
Ischium
Ischium
Radius
Carpal
Carpal
Metacarpal
Metacarpal
Pubis
Phalanx
Phalanx
Pubis
Femur
Femur
Patella
Knee joint
Knee joint
Tibia
Fibula
Fibula
Tibia
Ankle joint
Tarsal
Ankle joint
Tarsal
Metatarsal
Calcaneus
Metatarsal
Phalanx

FRONT VIEW

BACK VIEW

Skeleton varieties 2

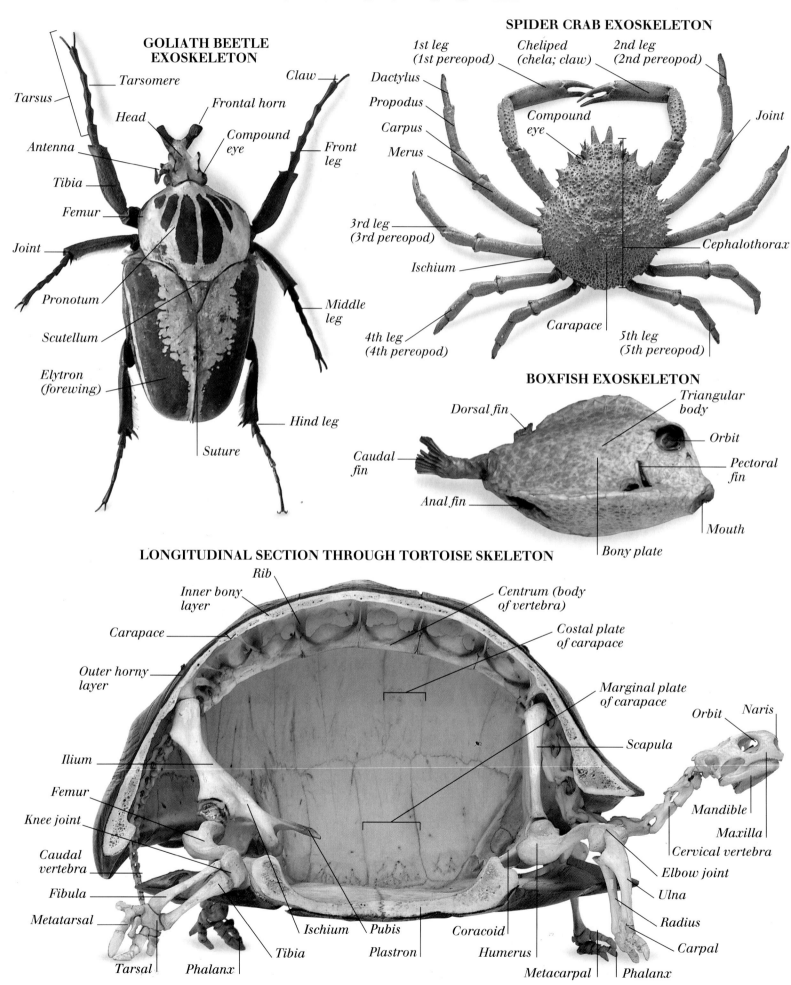

GOLIATH BEETLE EXOSKELETON

Tarsomere
Tarsus
Claw
Head
Frontal horn
Antenna
Compound eye
Front leg
Tibia
Femur
Joint
Pronotum
Scutellum
Middle leg
Elytron (forewing)
Hind leg
Suture

SPIDER CRAB EXOSKELETON

1st leg (1st pereopod)
Cheliped (chela; claw)
2nd leg (2nd pereopod)
Dactylus
Propodus
Compound eye
Joint
Carpus
Merus
3rd leg (3rd pereopod)
Cephalothorax
Ischium
Carapace
4th leg (4th pereopod)
5th leg (5th pereopod)

BOXFISH EXOSKELETON

Dorsal fin
Triangular body
Orbit
Caudal fin
Pectoral fin
Anal fin
Mouth
Bony plate

LONGITUDINAL SECTION THROUGH TORTOISE SKELETON

Rib
Inner bony layer
Centrum (body of vertebra)
Carapace
Costal plate of carapace
Outer horny layer
Marginal plate of carapace
Orbit
Naris
Ilium
Scapula
Femur
Knee joint
Caudal vertebra
Mandible
Maxilla
Cervical vertebra
Fibula
Elbow joint
Ulna
Metatarsal
Radius
Ischium
Pubis
Coracoid
Humerus
Carpal
Tarsal
Phalanx
Tibia
Plastron
Metacarpal
Phalanx

The human skeleton through life

THE SKELETON OF THE HUMAN FETUS is formed from tough but flexible cartilage that acts as a blueprint for bone construction. During ossification (changing to bone), which begins before birth, the cartilage is broken down and the resulting space is filled by bone-building mineral salts and protein fibers secreted by bone cells. At birth, the diaphyses (shafts) of the long bones are already ossified, while the epiphyses (ends of bones) are still cartilaginous. The epiphyses gradually ossify, leaving a cartilaginous epiphyseal plate (growth plate) where growth continues until late adolescence. The bones of the skull are formed by the ossification of fibrous tissue, rather than cartilage. In the newborn baby, this flexible tissue forms fontanelles between the partly ossified skull bones, allowing the cranium to enlarge as the brain grows. The facial bones also enlarge as the skull develops. After the age of about 40, bone mass starts to decrease, a process that is sometimes accelerated by osteoporosis.

GROWTH OF HUMAN SKULL

Sphenoidal fontanelle
Anterior fontanelle
Parietal bone
Frontal bone
Relatively large cranium
Orbit
Lambdoidal suture
Facial bones
Occipital bone
Maxilla
Mastoid fontanelle
Mandible
Zygomatic arch
Wide suture
Temporal bone

NEWBORN

Frontal bone
Parietal bone
Cranium approaching adult dimensions
Orbit
Facial bones enlarging
Narrowed suture easily visible
Deciduous (milk) tooth
Occipital bone
Erupting permanent tooth
Temporal bone
Mandible
Maxilla
Zygomatic arch

6 YEARS

PRIMARY OSSIFICATION CENTERS IN 12-WEEK-OLD FETUS

Parietal bone
Occipital bone
Frontal bone
Clavicle
Maxilla
Ossification begins at about 5 weeks
Phalanx
Scapula
Mandible
Ossification begins at about 6 to 8 weeks
Ulna
Humerus
Radius
Ossification begins at about 6 to 8 weeks
Ossification begins at about 6 to 16 weeks
Facial bones fully developed
Fibula
Maxilla
Rib
Tibia
Metacarpal
Phalanx
Hipbone
Mandible
Femur
Ossification begins at about 6 to 12 weeks
Ossification begins at about 6 to 12 weeks
Permanent tooth

Frontal bone
Supraorbital ridge
Parietal bone
Orbit
Cranium fully developed
Occipital bone
Suture closed up
Temporal bone
Zygomatic arch

ADULT

SEA URCHIN EXOSKELETON

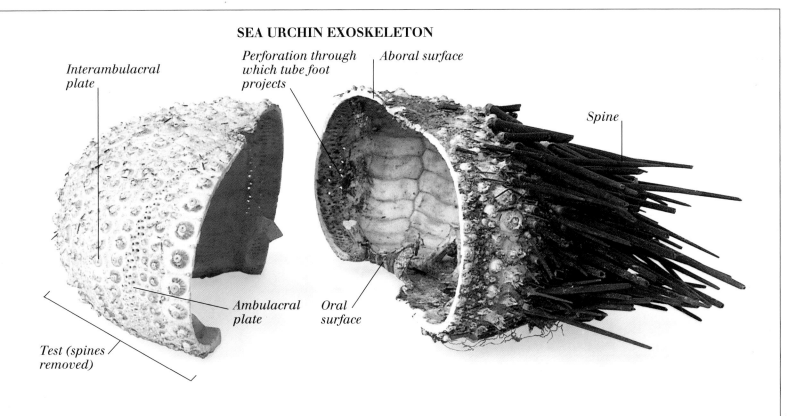

Interambulacral plate

Perforation through which tube foot projects

Aboral surface

Spine

Ambulacral plate

Oral surface

Test (spines removed)

DIATOM FRUSTULES

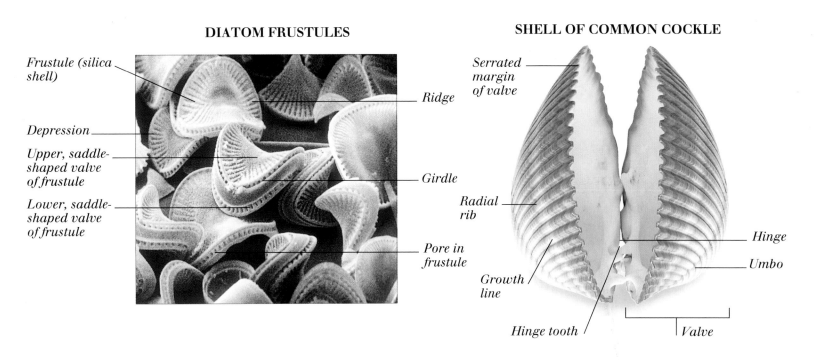

Frustule (silica shell)

Depression

Upper, saddle-shaped valve of frustule

Lower, saddle-shaped valve of frustule

Ridge

Girdle

Pore in frustule

SHELL OF COMMON COCKLE

Serrated margin of valve

Radial rib

Growth line

Hinge tooth

Hinge

Umbo

Valve

WORM HYDROSTATIC SKELETON

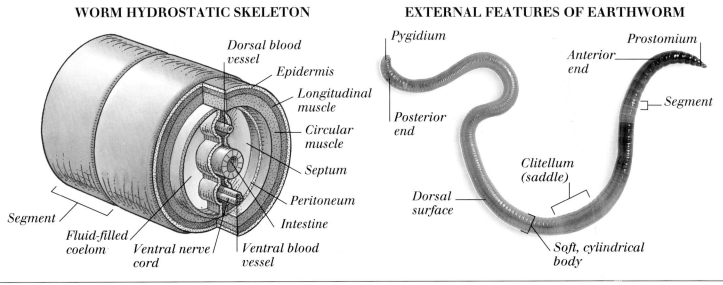

Dorsal blood vessel

Epidermis

Longitudinal muscle

Circular muscle

Septum

Peritoneum

Intestine

Ventral blood vessel

Segment

Fluid-filled coelom

Ventral nerve cord

EXTERNAL FEATURES OF EARTHWORM

Pygidium

Posterior end

Prostomium

Anterior end

Segment

Clitellum (saddle)

Dorsal surface

Soft, cylindrical body

BONE DEVELOPMENT IN HUMAN HAND

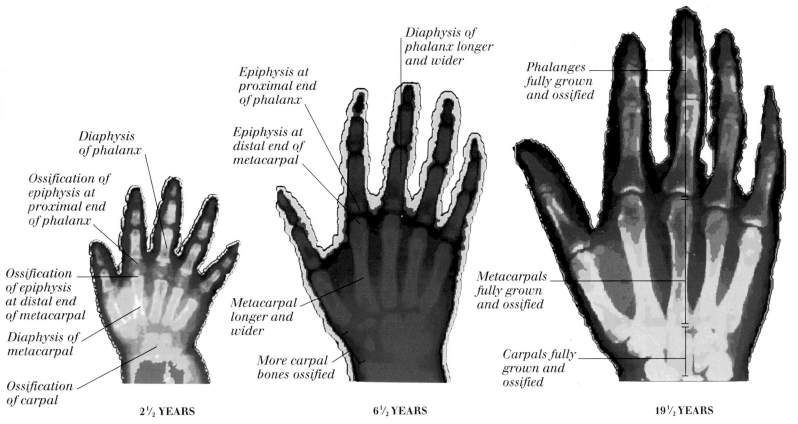

Diaphysis of phalanx

Ossification of epiphysis at proximal end of phalanx

Ossification of epiphysis at distal end of metacarpal

Diaphysis of metacarpal

Ossification of carpal

2½ YEARS

Epiphysis at proximal end of phalanx

Epiphysis at distal end of metacarpal

Diaphysis of phalanx longer and wider

Metacarpal longer and wider

More carpal bones ossified

6½ YEARS

Phalanges fully grown and ossified

Metacarpals fully grown and ossified

Carpals fully grown and ossified

19½ YEARS

SCANNING ELECTRON MICROGRAPH OF CANCELLOUS BONE

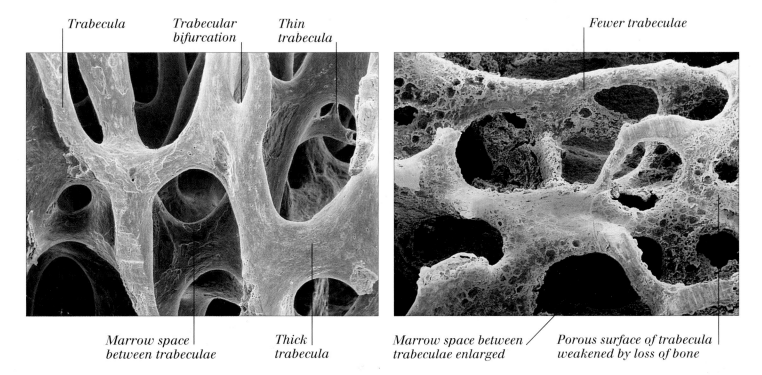

Trabecula

Trabecular bifurcation

Thin trabecula

Fewer trabeculae

Marrow space between trabeculae

Thick trabecula

Marrow space between trabeculae enlarged

Porous surface of trabecula weakened by loss of bone

HEALTHY BONE

BONE WITH OSTEOPOROSIS

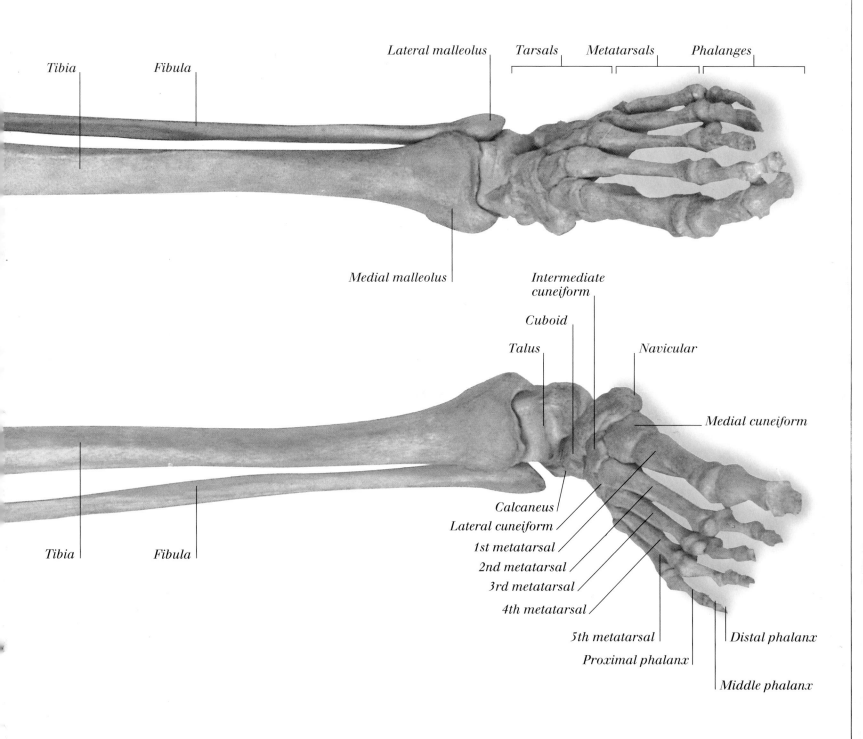

Tibia

Fibula

Lateral malleolus

Tarsals

Metatarsals

Phalanges

Medial malleolus

Intermediate
cuneiform

Cuboid

Talus

Navicular

Medial cuneiform

Calcaneus

Lateral cuneiform

1st metatarsal

2nd metatarsal

3rd metatarsal

4th metatarsal

5th metatarsal

Proximal phalanx

Distal phalanx

Middle phalanx

Tibia

Fibula

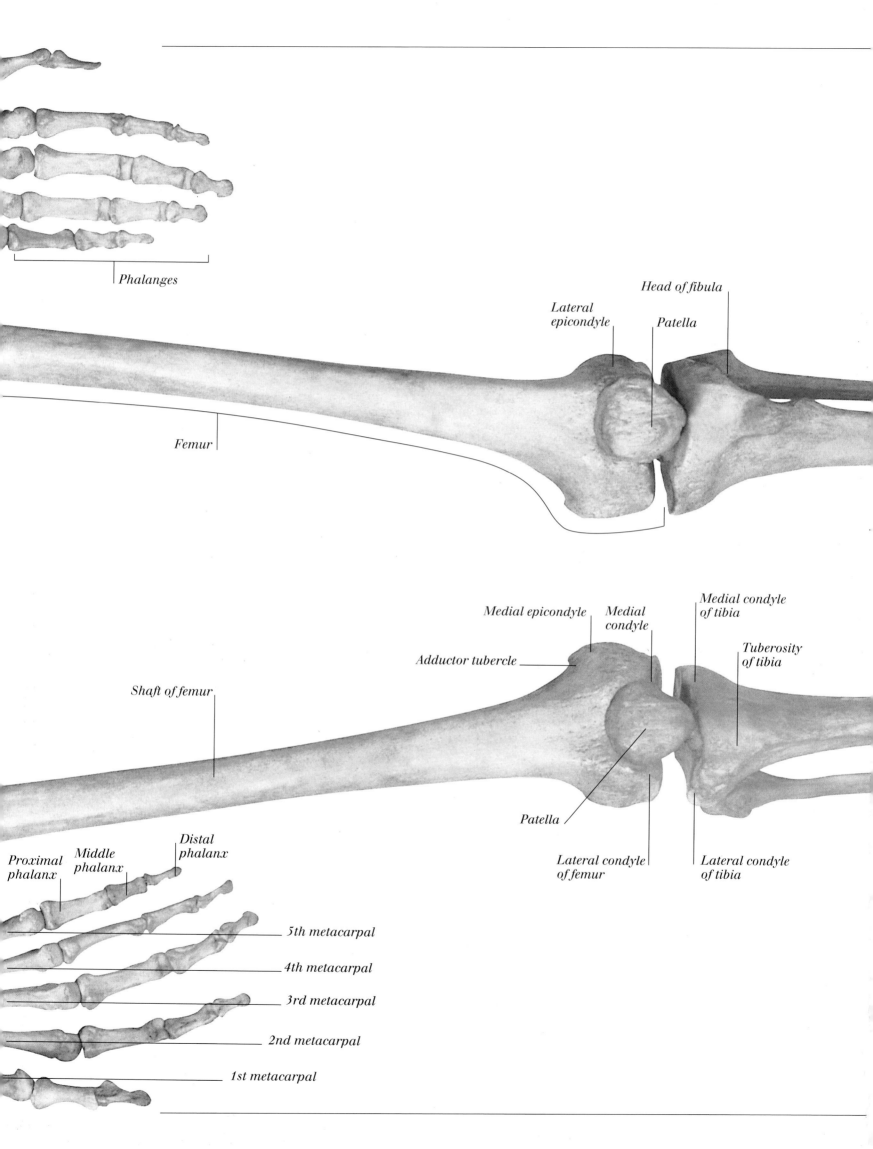

Phalanges

Femur

Shaft of femur

Proximal phalanx   Middle phalanx   Distal phalanx

5th metacarpal

4th metacarpal

3rd metacarpal

2nd metacarpal

1st metacarpal

Lateral epicondyle   Patella   Head of fibula

Medial epicondyle   Medial condyle   Medial condyle of tibia

Adductor tubercle

Tuberosity of tibia

Patella

Lateral condyle of femur   Lateral condyle of tibia

Plant skeletons

SKELETON OF
MAGNOLIA
LEAF

PLANTS TYPICALLY HAVE A STEM that bears leaves and flowers, and roots that anchor the plant in the soil. The stem and roots are supported and protected by a skeletal system. The skeleton of the stem helps the plant resist any bending that is caused by external forces; it also holds the leaves in position so that they can receive the sunlight necessary for photosynthesis. The stems of herbaceous (nonwoody) plants are supported by cells called sclerenchyma and collenchyma, and by strong-walled, water-conducting cells called xylem. In woody plants, the trunks and branches are supported by an inner core of xylem and associated fibers, which together form the wood. As the wood in the center of the tree gets older, it loses its conductive role but continues to support the stem. This nonconducting wood is known as heartwood. The outer, conducting wood is known as sapwood. Roots have a central cylinder of transport tissue, which is known as the stele. The stele contains tough xylem that enables roots to resist the pressure produced as they grow through the soil.

MICROGRAPH OF XYLEM IN BUTTERCUP STEM

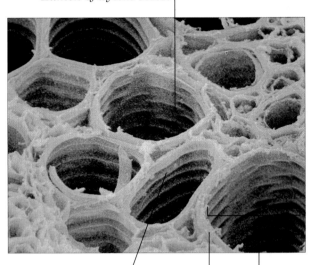

Lumen of xylem vessel

Annular thickening in wall of xylem vessel

Lignified cell wall of xylem vessel

Xylem vessel

LONGITUDINAL SECTION THROUGH BUTTERCUP ROOT

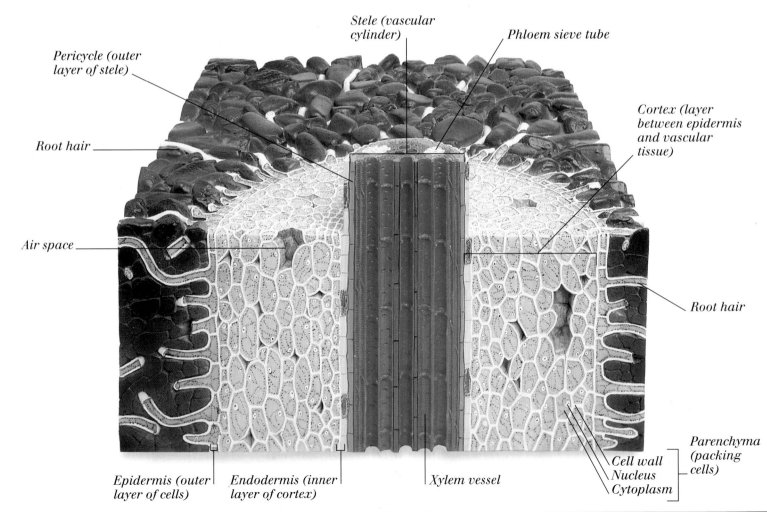

Stele (vascular cylinder)

Phloem sieve tube

Pericycle (outer layer of stele)

Cortex (layer between epidermis and vascular tissue)

Root hair

Air space

Root hair

Epidermis (outer layer of cells)

Endodermis (inner layer of cortex)

Xylem vessel

Cell wall

Nucleus

Cytoplasm

Parenchyma (packing cells)

TREE SHOWING EXTERNAL STRESSES

Heavy rainfall and snow

Strong winds

Weight of leaves in summer

Pressure as root pushes through earth

Roots act as anchors and resist pulling forces that result from movement above ground

CROSS-SECTION THROUGH MATURE STEM OF BISHOP PINE

Sapwood (active secondary xylem)

Annual ring

Heartwood (inactive secondary xylem)

Branch trace (vascular bundle supplying branch)

Pith

Bark
- Phloem
- Periderm

LONGITUDINAL SECTION THROUGH YOUNG WOODY STEM

Secondary phloem

Cortex (layer between phellem and vascular tissue)

Xylem vessel

Xylem fiber (supporting tissue)

Ray (parenchyma cells)

Phloem sieve tube

Phloem fiber (supporting tissue)

Lenticel (pore)

Phellem (protective cork layer)

Pith

Vascular cambium (actively dividing cells that produce xylem and phloem)

Autumn wood

Spring wood

Secondary xylem

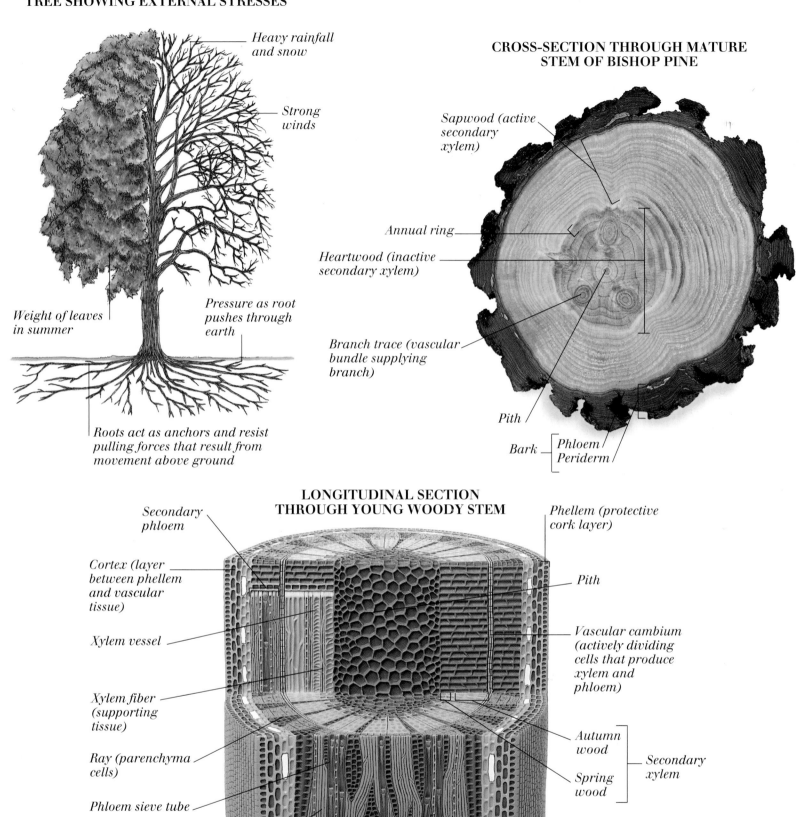

Shells and simple skeletons

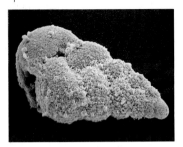

FOSSIL FORAMINIFERAN

SHELLS ARE EXOSKELETONS that protect the soft bodies of most mollusks. Each mollusk group has a characteristic shell form. Gastropods, such as the lightning whelk, have a cone-shaped, spiral shell, made up of tubular whorls, with an aperture through which the animal's head is extended or retracted. Bivalves, such as the mussel, have a hinged shell with two halves that are opened and closed by powerful muscles. Cephalopods, such as the octopus, generally lack external shells. However, one cephalopod, *Nautilus*, has a flattened spiral shell, divided into chambers. The animal occupies only the body chamber. Some other invertebrates have simple exoskeletons. Corals, for example, are colonial invertebrates that build protective calcium carbonate cases into which they can retreat. Foraminiferans are aquatic protozoans with a shell that protects their amoeboid body.

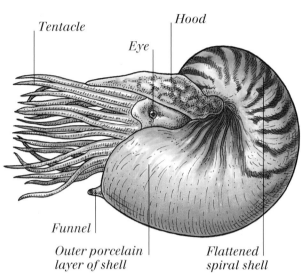

Tentacle

Eye

Hood

Funnel

Outer porcelain layer of shell

Flattened spiral shell

SECTION THROUGH NAUTILUS SHELL

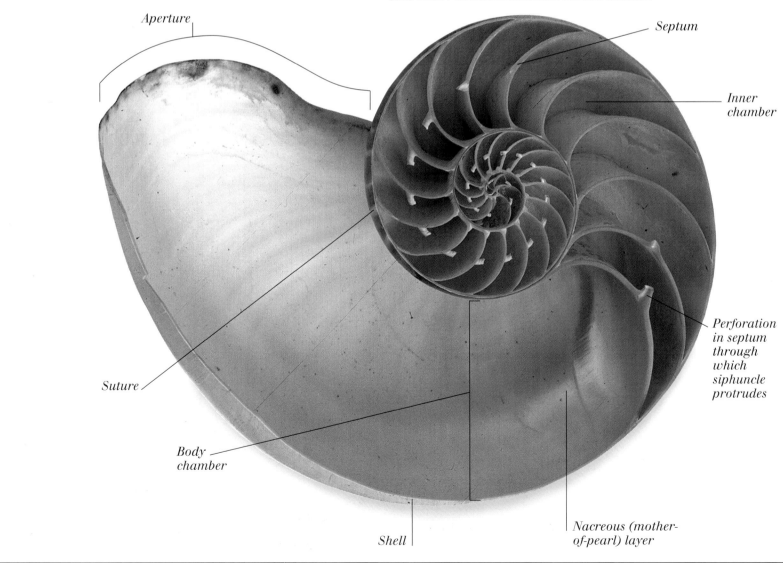

Aperture

Septum

Inner chamber

Perforation in septum through which siphuncle protrudes

Suture

Body chamber

Nacreous (mother-of-pearl) layer

Shell

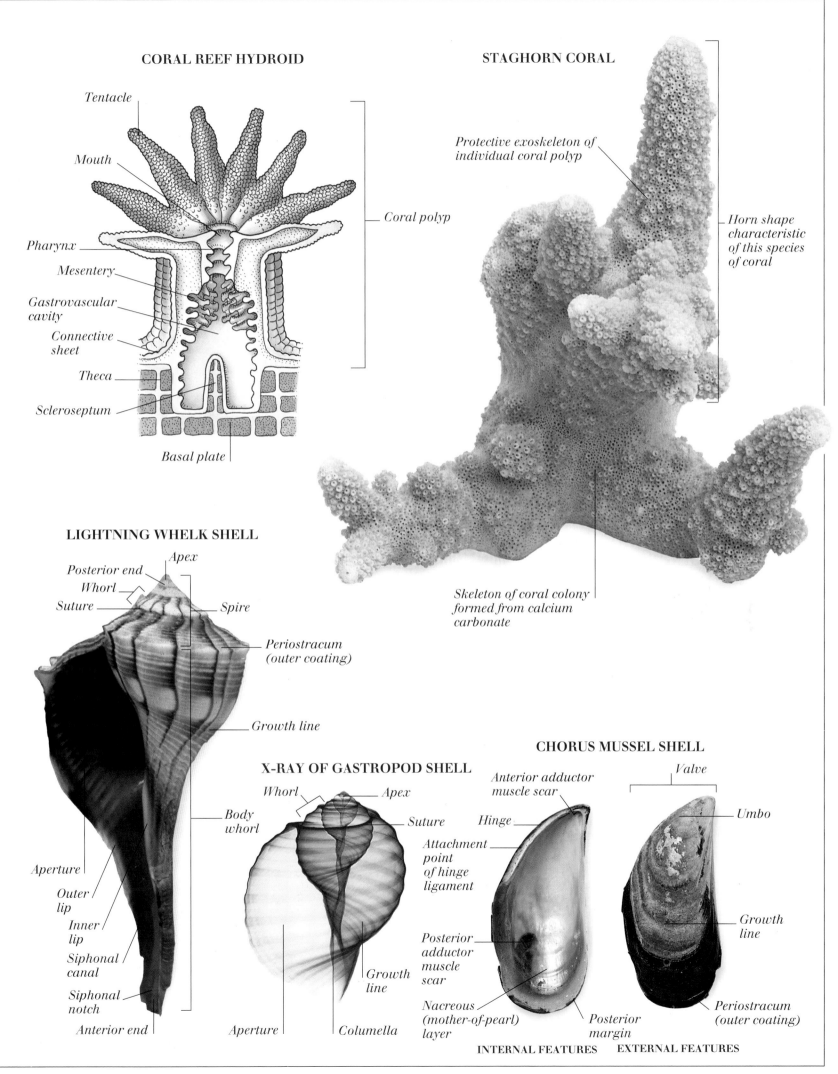

CORAL REEF HYDROID

Tentacle

Mouth

Coral polyp

Pharynx

Mesentery

Gastrovascular cavity

Connective sheet

Theca

Scleroseptum

Basal plate

STAGHORN CORAL

Protective exoskeleton of individual coral polyp

Horn shape characteristic of this species of coral

Skeleton of coral colony formed from calcium carbonate

LIGHTNING WHELK SHELL

Apex

Posterior end

Whorl

Suture

Spire

Periostracum (outer coating)

Growth line

Body whorl

Aperture

Outer lip

Inner lip

Siphonal canal

Siphonal notch

Anterior end

X-RAY OF GASTROPOD SHELL

Whorl

Apex

Suture

Growth line

Aperture

Columella

CHORUS MUSSEL SHELL

Valve

Anterior adductor muscle scar

Hinge

Umbo

Attachment point of hinge ligament

Posterior adductor muscle scar

Growth line

Nacreous (mother-of-pearl) layer

Posterior margin

Periostracum (outer coating)

INTERNAL FEATURES

EXTERNAL FEATURES

Arthropod exoskeletons

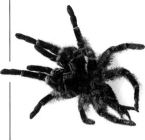

TARANTULA MOLT

MOST ANIMALS WITH exoskeletons belong to the arthropod group (animals with jointed limbs), which includes insects, such as beetles; arachnids, such as scorpions; and crustaceans, such as crabs. The arthropod exoskeleton, also known as the cuticle, encases the entire body (including the eyes), and consists of inflexible plates that meet at flexible joints. The joints are formed by thinner sections of cuticle called articular membranes. Muscles, attached to the exoskeleton across these joints, contract to produce movement. The arthropod exoskeleton cannot expand, and must be molted periodically to allow the animal to grow. An exoskeleton also imposes a maximum size on arthropods: although the cuticle contains a substance called chitin that makes it both hard and light, above a certain body size the cuticle becomes so heavy that movement is impossible.

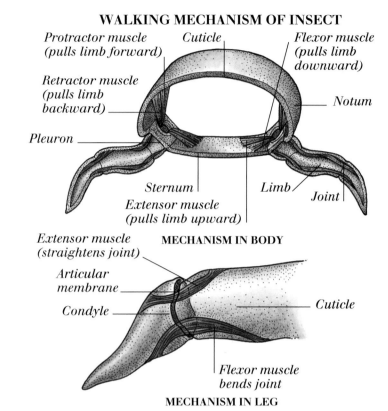

WALKING MECHANISM OF INSECT

Protractor muscle (pulls limb forward)
Cuticle
Flexor muscle (pulls limb downward)
Retractor muscle (pulls limb backward)
Notum
Pleuron
Sternum
Limb
Joint
Extensor muscle (pulls limb upward)

MECHANISM IN BODY

Extensor muscle (straightens joint)
Articular membrane
Cuticle
Condyle
Flexor muscle bends joint

MECHANISM IN LEG

SCORPION EXOSKELETON

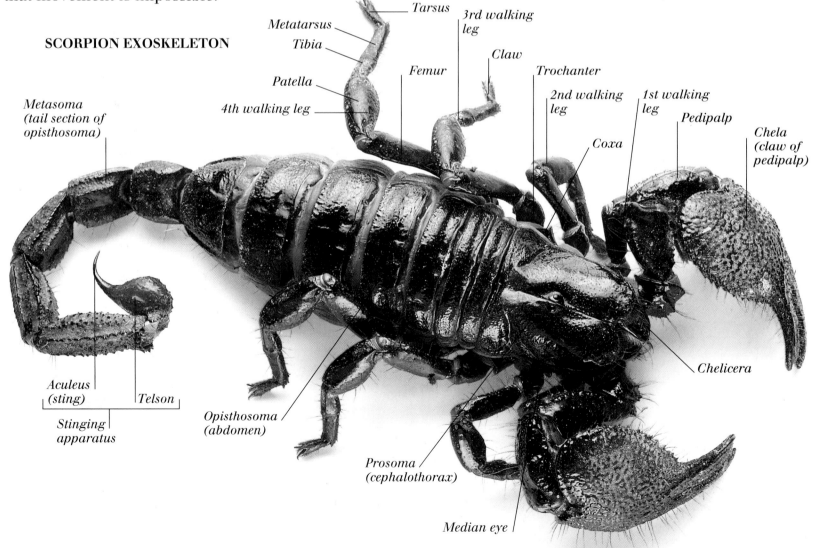

Tarsus
Metatarsus
3rd walking leg
Tibia
Claw
Femur
Trochanter
Patella
2nd walking leg
1st walking leg
4th walking leg
Pedipalp
Chela (claw of pedipalp)
Metasoma (tail section of opisthosoma)
Coxa
Chelicera
Aculeus (sting)
Telson
Stinging apparatus
Opisthosoma (abdomen)
Prosoma (cephalothorax)
Median eye

CRAB EXOSKELETON

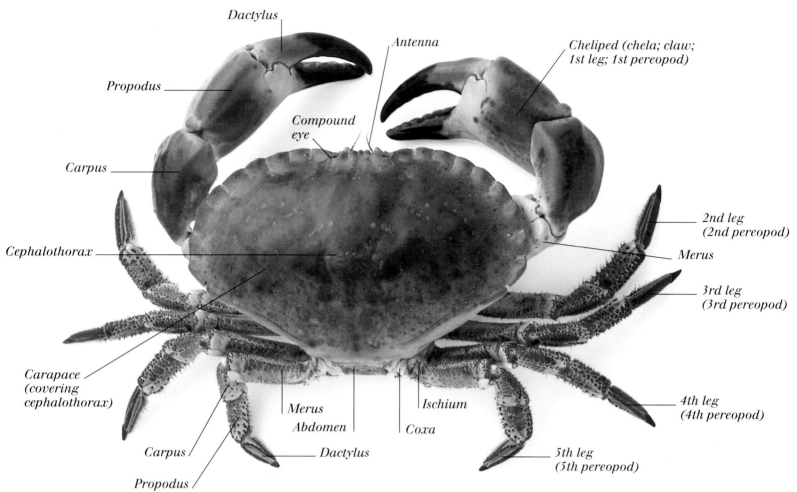

Dactylus

Propodus

Antenna

Cheliped (chela; claw; 1st leg; 1st pereopod)

Compound eye

Carpus

Cephalothorax

Carapace (covering cephalothorax)

Merus

Abdomen

Carpus

Propodus

Dactylus

Ischium

Coxa

2nd leg (2nd pereopod)

Merus

3rd leg (3rd pereopod)

4th leg (4th pereopod)

5th leg (5th pereopod)

FLYING MECHANISM OF INSECT

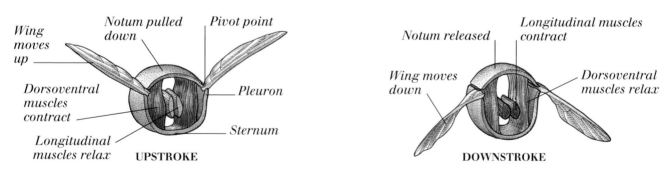

Wing moves up

Notum pulled down

Pivot point

Dorsoventral muscles contract

Pleuron

Longitudinal muscles relax

Sternum

UPSTROKE

Notum released

Longitudinal muscles contract

Wing moves down

Dorsoventral muscles relax

DOWNSTROKE

EXOSKELETON OF MALE ATLAS BEETLE

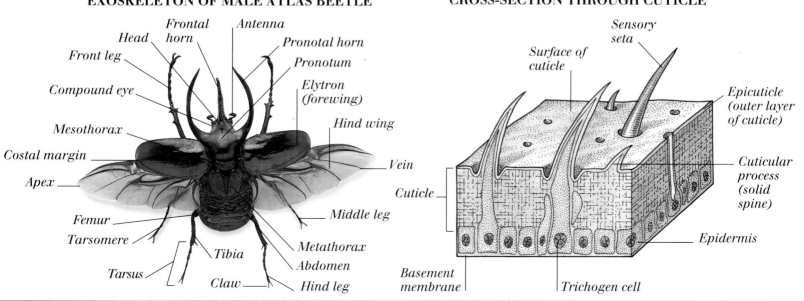

Frontal horn

Antenna

Head

Pronotal horn

Front leg

Pronotum

Compound eye

Elytron (forewing)

Mesothorax

Hind wing

Costal margin

Apex

Vein

Femur

Middle leg

Tarsomere

Metathorax

Tarsus

Tibia

Abdomen

Claw

Hind leg

CROSS-SECTION THROUGH CUTICLE

Sensory seta

Surface of cuticle

Epicuticle (outer layer of cuticle)

Cuticle

Cuticular process (solid spine)

Epidermis

Basement membrane

Trichogen cell

Fish skeletons

FISHES WERE THE FIRST VERTEBRATES to evolve, and the first animals to have endoskeletons (internal skeletons). Bony fishes, such as cod and salmon, have a skeleton that is made of bone, as do most other vertebrates. Cartilaginous fishes, such as sharks (including dogfish) and rays, have a skeleton made of cartilage: a strong, flexible material that is also found in the human ear and nose. The fish skeleton produces a streamlined shape, adapting the animal for movement in water. It also has fins for propelling, stabilizing, and steering. The taperered skull minimizes drag as the fish moves forward, and supports and protects the brain and gills. The flexible vertebral column (backbone) has muscles attached on either side along its length. These muscles contract alternately, bending the body from side to side to propel the fish forward through the water. The fins, including the tail, are supported by bones and rods. The dorsal and ventral fins, positioned on the midline, prevent the fish from rolling; the paired pectoral and pelvic fins allow it to control its direction.

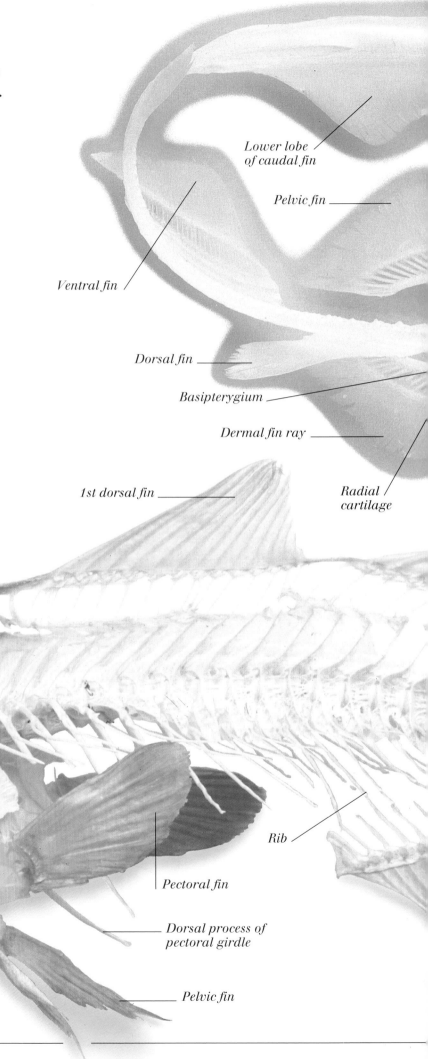

Lower lobe of caudal fin

Pelvic fin

Ventral fin

Dorsal fin

Basipterygium

Dermal fin ray

1st dorsal fin

Radial cartilage

COD SKELETON

Opercular bone

Supraoccipital bone

Postparietal bone

COD

Preopercular bone

Hyomandibular bone

Orbit

Parietal bone

Lacrimal bone

Maxilla

Frontal bone

Rib

Pectoral fin

Dorsal process of pectoral girdle

Subopercular bone

Pelvic fin

Dentary bone

Quadrate bone

Premaxilla

Articular bone

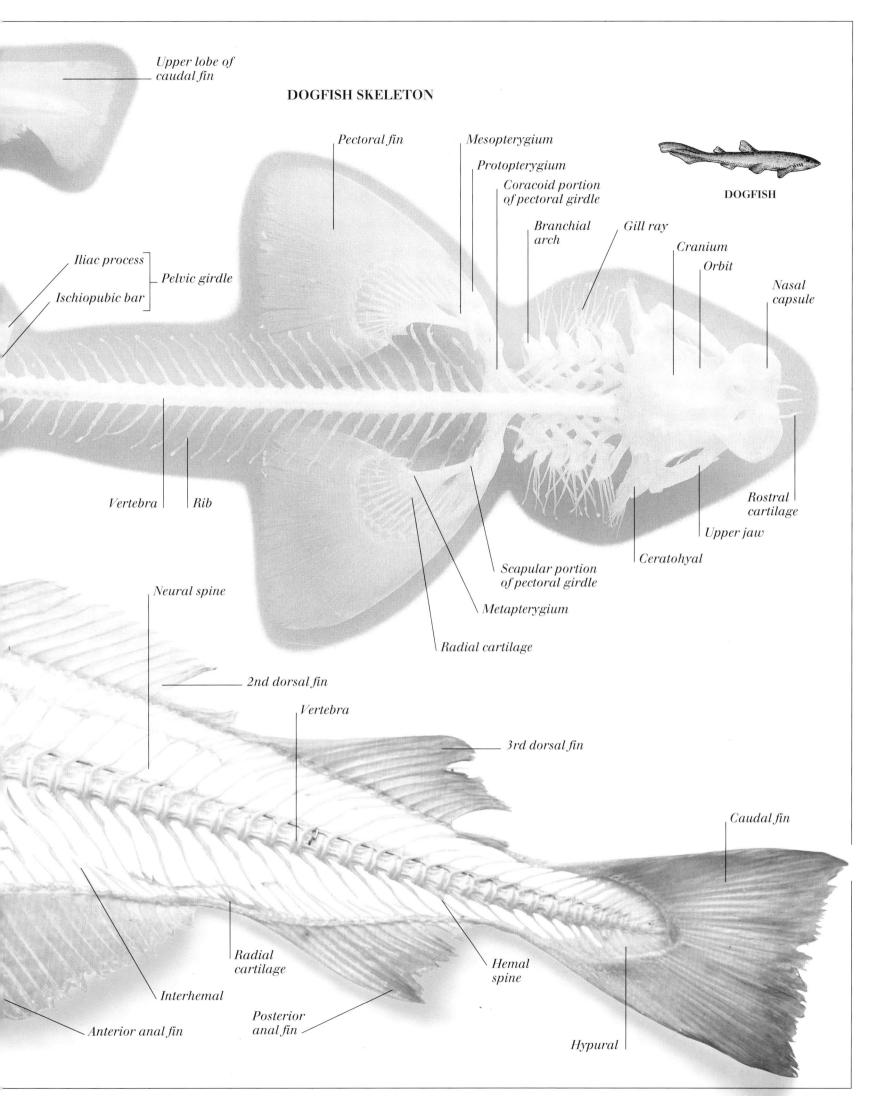

Upper lobe of
caudal fin

DOGFISH SKELETON

Pectoral fin

Mesopterygium

Protopterygium

Coracoid portion
of pectoral girdle

Branchial
arch

Gill ray

Cranium

Orbit

DOGFISH

Nasal
capsule

Iliac process

Ischiopubic bar

Pelvic girdle

Vertebra

Rib

Scapular portion
of pectoral girdle

Metapterygium

Radial cartilage

Rostral
cartilage

Upper jaw

Ceratohyal

Neural spine

2nd dorsal fin

Vertebra

3rd dorsal fin

Caudal fin

Radial
cartilage

Hemal
spine

Interhemal

Anterior anal fin

Posterior
anal fin

Hypural

Amphibian skeletons

AMPHIBIANS ARE VERTEBRATES that typically are adapted for life both on land and in water. Most amphibians have a bony endoskeleton, although some species of salamander have mainly cartilaginous pectoral (shoulder) and pelvic (hip) girdles. The three amphibian groups show considerable skeletal variation. Frogs and toads have a short, squat body; a broad skull with a wide mouth and large orbits; and long hind limbs and feet for jumping and swimming. The large pelvic girdle transmits force from the hind legs to the rest of the body through a short, inflexible backbone. The pectoral girdle is generally strengthened to withstand the force of landing. Salamanders have elongated bodies with tails; a flexible backbone that curves from side to side during movement on land or in water; short front and hind legs; and a broad skull. The third amphibian group, the caecilians, are adapted for burrowing. Their limbless skeletons have a compact skull with no orbits, and a long, flexible backbone with up to 100 vertebrae.

SALAMANDER SKELETON

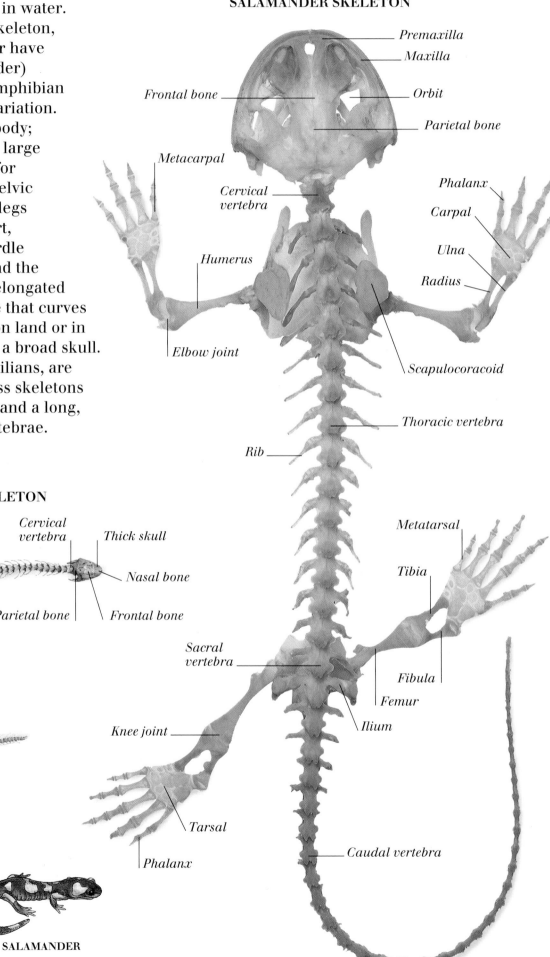

Premaxilla

Maxilla

Frontal bone

Orbit

Parietal bone

Metacarpal

Cervical vertebra

Phalanx

Carpal

Humerus

Ulna

Radius

Elbow joint

Scapulocoracoid

Thoracic vertebra

Rib

Metatarsal

Tibia

Sacral vertebra

Fibula

Femur

Knee joint

Ilium

Tarsal

Caudal vertebra

Phalanx

CAECILIAN SKELETON

Rib

Cervical vertebra

Thick skull

Nasal bone

Vertebra

Parietal bone

Frontal bone

CAECILIAN

SALAMANDER

FROG SKELETON

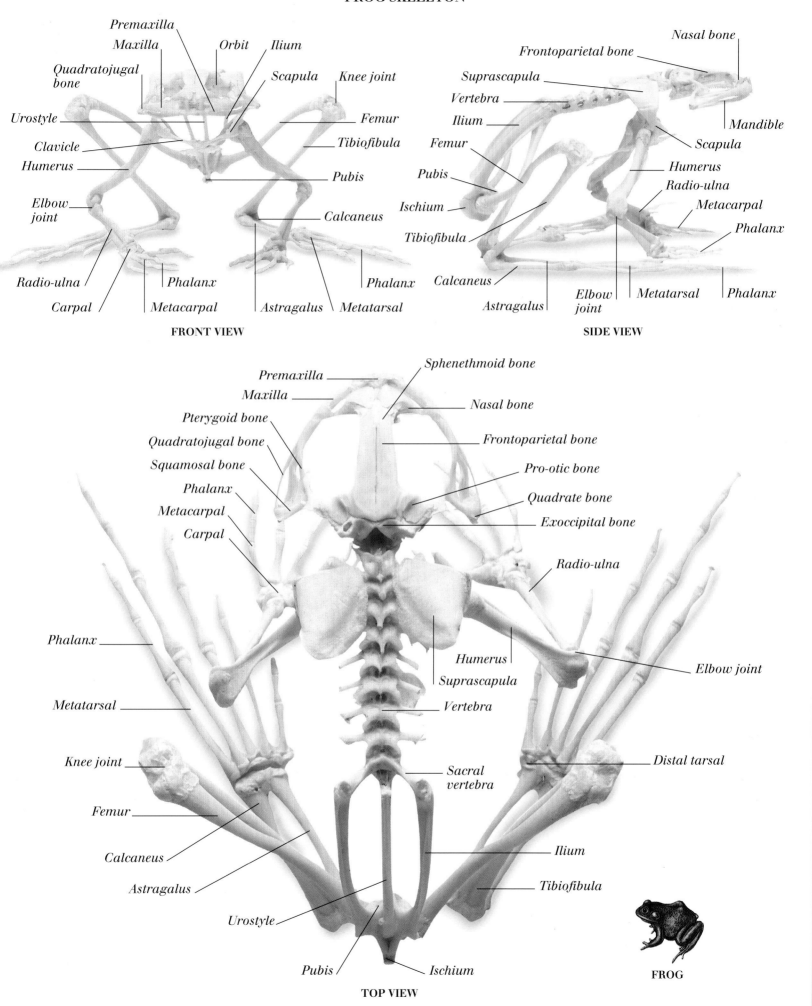

FRONT VIEW

Premaxilla
Maxilla
Quadratojugal bone
Orbit
Ilium
Scapula
Knee joint
Urostyle
Femur
Clavicle
Tibiofibula
Humerus
Pubis
Elbow joint
Calcaneus
Radio-ulna
Phalanx
Carpal
Metacarpal
Astragalus
Metatarsal
Phalanx

SIDE VIEW

Frontoparietal bone
Nasal bone
Suprascapula
Vertebra
Ilium
Mandible
Scapula
Femur
Humerus
Pubis
Radio-ulna
Ischium
Metacarpal
Tibiofibula
Phalanx
Calcaneus
Elbow joint
Metatarsal
Phalanx
Astragalus

TOP VIEW

Premaxilla
Sphenethmoid bone
Maxilla
Pterygoid bone
Nasal bone
Quadratojugal bone
Frontoparietal bone
Squamosal bone
Pro-otic bone
Phalanx
Quadrate bone
Metacarpal
Exoccipital bone
Carpal
Radio-ulna
Phalanx
Humerus
Suprascapula
Elbow joint
Metatarsal
Vertebra
Knee joint
Sacral vertebra
Distal tarsal
Femur
Calcaneus
Ilium
Astragalus
Tibiofibula
Urostyle
Pubis
Ischium

FROG

Reptile skeletons 1

REPTILES ARE VERTEBRATES with a bony endoskeleton. Typically, the reptile skeleton is elongated, with a flexible backbone, and short legs that project sideways. However, skeletal variations occur within the group. For example, snakes lack limbs but have a long backbone consisting of between about 180 and 400 vertebrae. Snakes also have a highly flexible jaw mechanism, allowing large prey to be swallowed whole. Turtles have both an exoskeleton and an endoskeleton. The exoskeleton consists of a shell with an outer, horny layer and an inner, bony layer. The ribs, backbone, and pectoral (shoulder) and pelvic (hip) girdles of the endoskeleton are fused to the inner layer of the exoskeleton. Crocodilians, such as the gharial and the Nile crocodile, are semiaquatic reptiles with a long tail for swimming; a long snout with pointed teeth; and nostrils and eye sockets set high on the skull. Lizards generally follow the typical reptile body plan, but many also have features adapted to their environment, such as the tree-dwelling chameleon, which has opposable toes and a prehensile tail for grasping branches. Lizardlike tuataras retain primitive reptilian features, such as two complete temporal fenestrae (openings in the skull) and teeth that are fused to the jaw.

SNAKE SKELETON

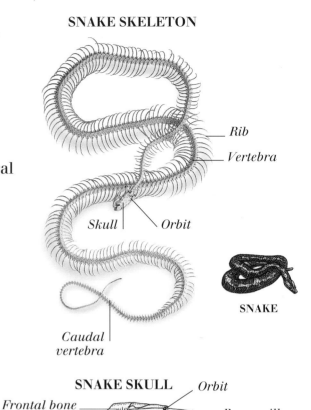

Rib

Vertebra

Skull

Orbit

SNAKE

Caudal vertebra

SNAKE SKULL

Orbit

Frontal bone

Premaxilla

Parietal bone

Maxilla

Supratemporal bone

Postfrontal bone

Quadrate bone

Ectopterygoid bone

Pterygoid bone

Articular bone

Surangular bone

Dentary bone

GHARIAL SKULL

Articular bone

Parietal bone

Squamosal bone

Infratemporal fenestra

Quadrate bone

Frontal bone

Postorbital bone

Orbit

Maxilla

Premaxilla

Jugal bone

Surangular bone

Angular bone

Mandibular fenestra

Dentary bone

Mandible

Naris

GHARIAL

Caudal vertebrae

Lumbar vertebrae

Sacrum

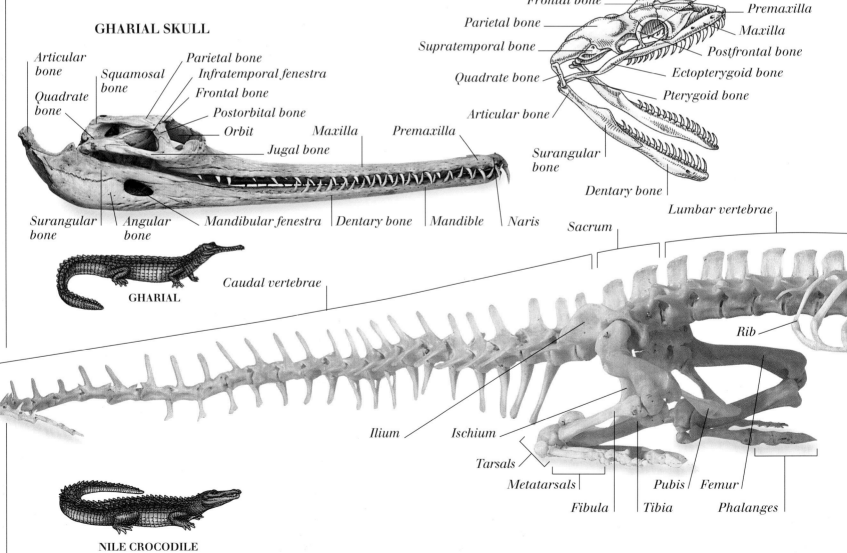

Rib

Ilium

Ischium

Tarsals

Metatarsals

Pubis

Femur

Fibula

Tibia

Phalanges

NILE CROCODILE

TURTLE SKELETON

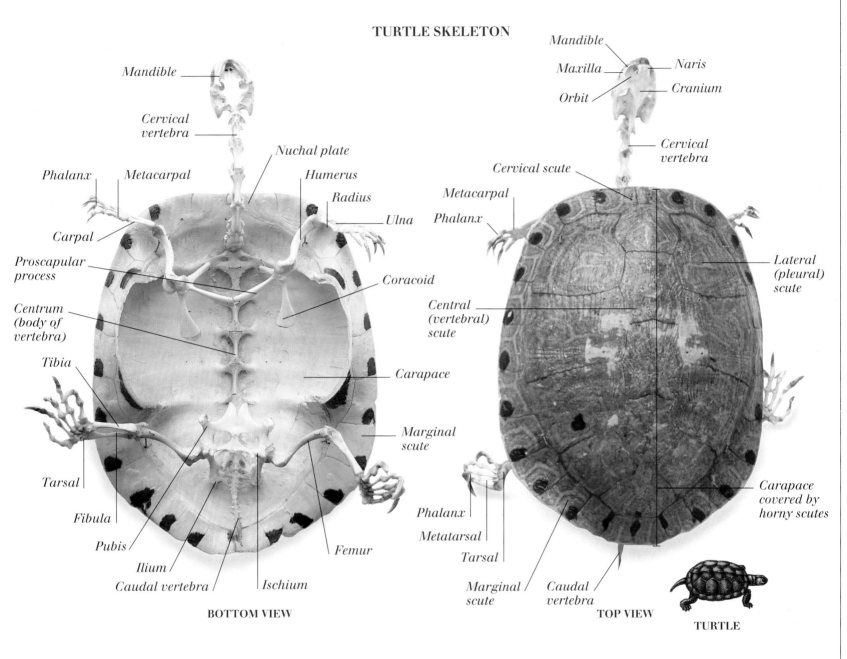

Mandible

Cervical vertebra

Phalanx

Metacarpal

Nuchal plate

Humerus

Radius

Ulna

Carpal

Proscapular process

Coracoid

Centrum (body of vertebra)

Tibia

Carapace

Tarsal

Marginal scute

Fibula

Pubis

Ilium

Caudal vertebra

Ischium

Femur

BOTTOM VIEW

Mandible

Maxilla

Naris

Orbit

Cranium

Cervical vertebra

Cervical scute

Metacarpal

Phalanx

Lateral (pleural) scute

Central (vertebral) scute

Carapace covered by horny scutes

Phalanx

Metatarsal

Tarsal

Marginal scute

Caudal vertebra

TOP VIEW

TURTLE

NILE CROCODILE SKELETON

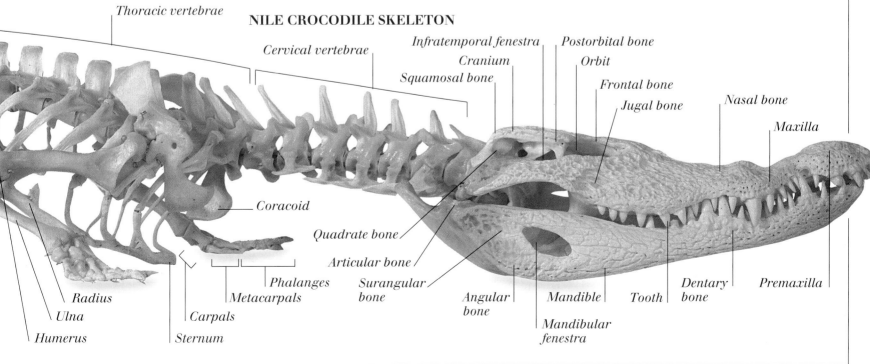

Thoracic vertebrae

Cervical vertebrae

Infratemporal fenestra

Postorbital bone

Cranium

Orbit

Squamosal bone

Frontal bone

Jugal bone

Nasal bone

Maxilla

Coracoid

Quadrate bone

Articular bone

Surangular bone

Angular bone

Mandible

Tooth

Dentary bone

Premaxilla

Phalanges

Metacarpals

Carpals

Sternum

Mandibular fenestra

Radius

Ulna

Humerus

Reptile skeletons 2

MONITOR LIZARD SKELETON

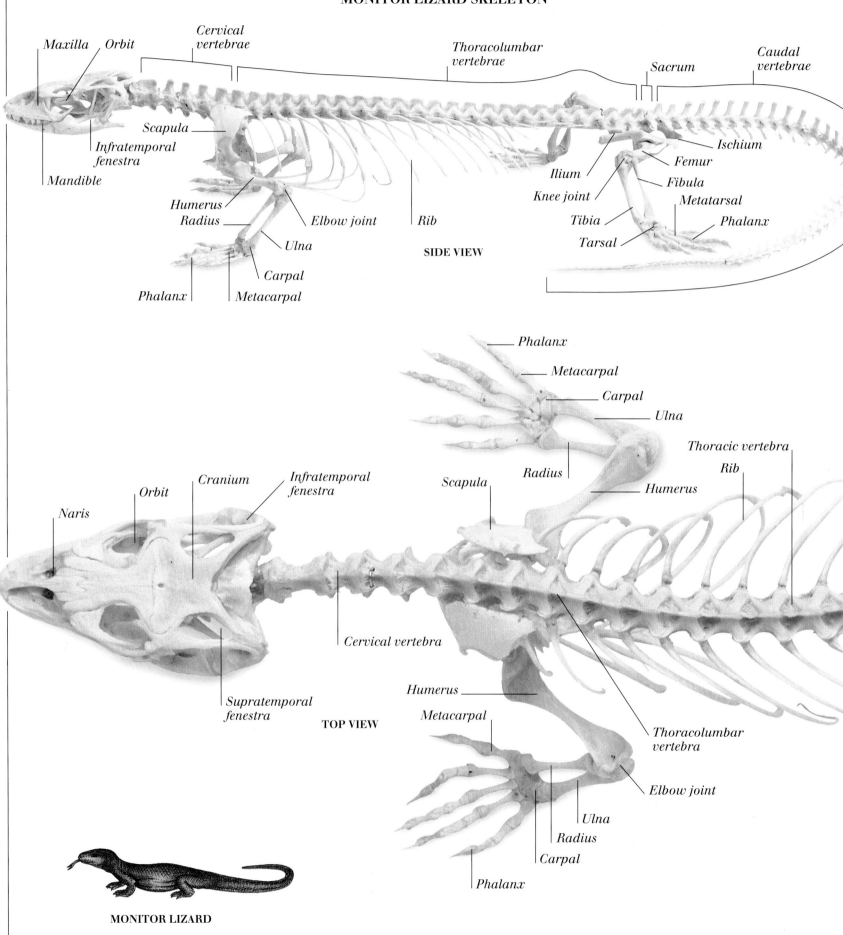

Maxilla *Orbit* *Cervical vertebrae* *Thoracolumbar vertebrae* *Sacrum* *Caudal vertebrae*

Scapula

Infratemporal fenestra

Mandible

Ischium

Femur

Ilium *Fibula*

Knee joint

Humerus *Metatarsal*

Radius *Elbow joint* *Rib* *Tibia* *Phalanx*

Ulna *Tarsal*

SIDE VIEW

Carpal

Phalanx *Metacarpal*

Phalanx

Metacarpal

Carpal

Ulna

Thoracic vertebra

Rib

Radius

Naris *Orbit* *Cranium* *Infratemporal fenestra* *Scapula* *Humerus*

Cervical vertebra

Supratemporal fenestra

Humerus

Thoracolumbar vertebra

Metacarpal

TOP VIEW

Elbow joint

Ulna

Radius

Carpal

Phalanx

MONITOR LIZARD

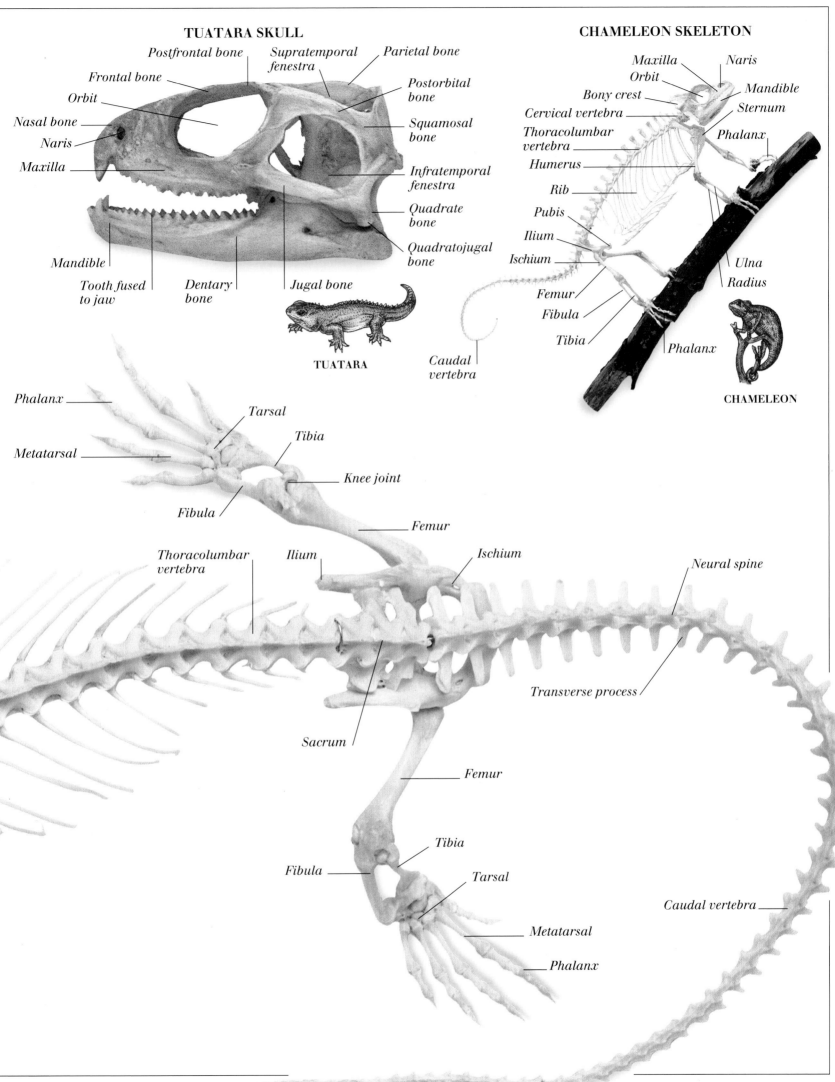

TUATARA SKULL

Postfrontal bone

Frontal bone

Supratemporal fenestra

Parietal bone

Orbit

Postorbital bone

Nasal bone

Squamosal bone

Naris

Maxilla

Infratemporal fenestra

Quadrate bone

Quadratojugal bone

Mandible

Tooth fused to jaw

Dentary bone

Jugal bone

TUATARA

CHAMELEON SKELETON

Maxilla

Naris

Orbit

Mandible

Bony crest

Sternum

Cervical vertebra

Thoracolumbar vertebra

Phalanx

Humerus

Rib

Pubis

Ilium

Ischium

Ulna

Radius

Femur

Fibula

Phalanx

Tibia

Caudal vertebra

CHAMELEON

Phalanx

Tarsal

Metatarsal

Tibia

Knee joint

Fibula

Femur

Thoracolumbar vertebra

Ilium

Ischium

Neural spine

Sacrum

Transverse process

Femur

Fibula

Tibia

Tarsal

Caudal vertebra

Metatarsal

Phalanx

Bird skeletons

MOST BIRDS HAVE SKELETONS ADAPTED for flight. The majority of these adaptations serve to make the skeleton lighter; they include hollow bones strengthened with struts; the fusing of some bones, such as the tarsometatarsus; a lightweight, horny bill instead of a heavy jawbone and teeth; forelimbs modified to form wings; and a sternum (breastbone) enlarged to form a central keel to which the powerful flight muscles—the pectoralis and supracoracoideus—are attached. The vertebral column (backbone) is also relatively short to increase stability during flight. Birds have resilient legs that provide support, enable them to walk, push the body off the ground at takeoff, and absorb most of the force of landing. The skeletons of flightless birds show adaptations for different types of movement. For example, the penguin is well adapted for aquatic life by having forelimbs and hind limbs that are modified for swimming underwater.

BONE STRUCTURE

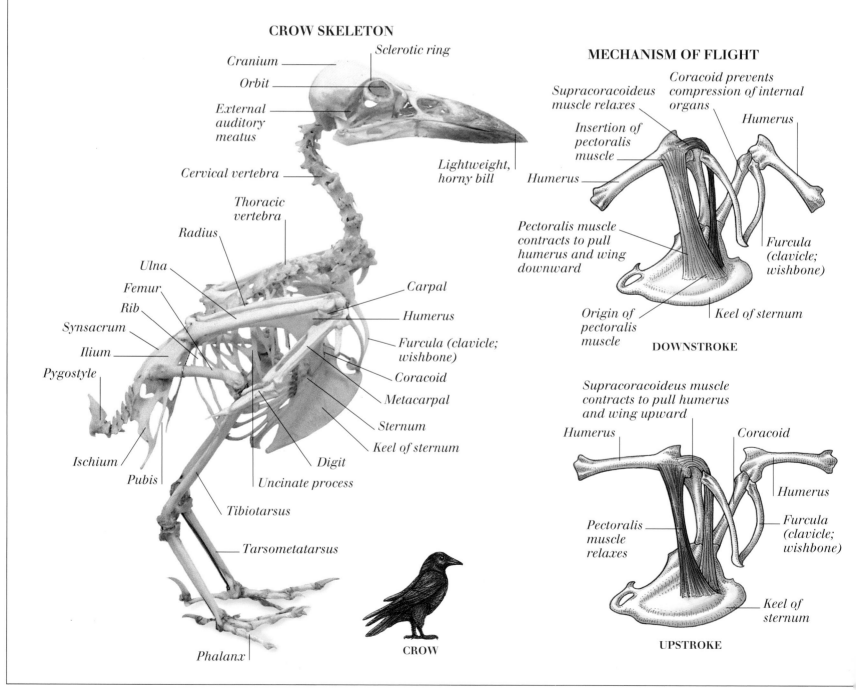

Lightweight, honeycombed interior

Bifurcation

Supporting strut

Air-filled space

WING BONE

Dense, honeycombed interior

Supporting strut

Bifurcation

Air-filled space

SKULL BONE

CROW SKELETON

Cranium

Sclerotic ring

Orbit

External auditory meatus

Lightweight, horny bill

Cervical vertebra

Thoracic vertebra

Radius

Ulna

Femur

Rib

Synsacrum

Ilium

Pygostyle

Ischium

Pubis

Tibiotarsus

Tarsometatarsus

Carpal

Humerus

Furcula (clavicle; wishbone)

Coracoid

Metacarpal

Sternum

Keel of sternum

Digit

Uncinate process

Phalanx

CROW

MECHANISM OF FLIGHT

Coracoid prevents compression of internal organs

Supracoracoideus muscle relaxes

Insertion of pectoralis muscle

Humerus

Humerus

Pectoralis muscle contracts to pull humerus and wing downward

Furcula (clavicle; wishbone)

Origin of pectoralis muscle

Keel of sternum

DOWNSTROKE

Supracoracoideus muscle contracts to pull humerus and wing upward

Humerus

Coracoid

Pectoralis muscle relaxes

Humerus

Furcula (clavicle; wishbone)

Keel of sternum

UPSTROKE

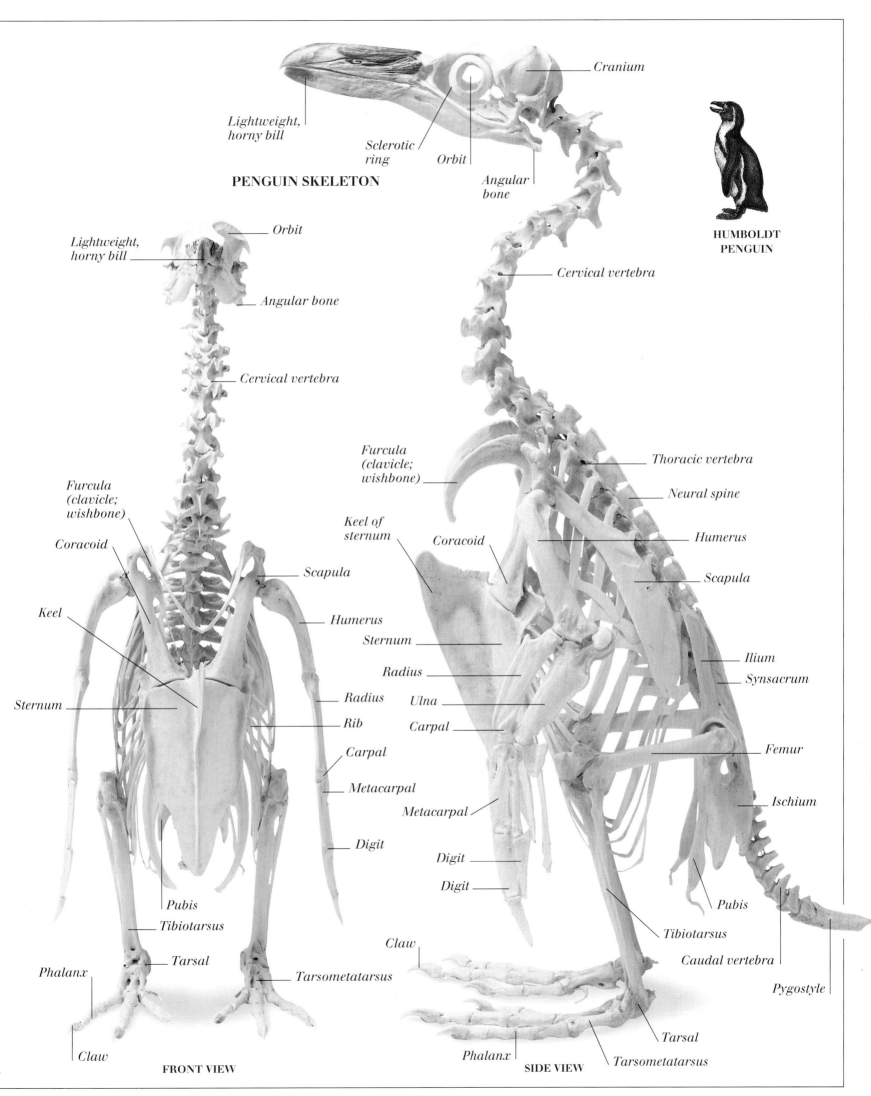

PENGUIN SKELETON

Lightweight, horny bill

Sclerotic ring

Orbit

Cranium

Angular bone

HUMBOLDT PENGUIN

Orbit

Lightweight, horny bill

Angular bone

Cervical vertebra

Cervical vertebra

Furcula (clavicle; wishbone)

Thoracic vertebra

Neural spine

Keel of sternum

Coracoid

Humerus

Furcula (clavicle; wishbone)

Coracoid

Scapula

Keel

Scapula

Humerus

Sternum

Radius

Ilium

Synsacrum

Sternum

Radius

Ulna

Rib

Carpal

Carpal

Metacarpal

Femur

Metacarpal

Ischium

Digit

Digit

Pubis

Digit

Tibiotarsus

Pubis

Claw

Caudal vertebra

Tarsal

Tarsometatarsus

Tibiotarsus

Pygostyle

Phalanx

Claw

Phalanx

Tarsal

Tarsometatarsus

FRONT VIEW

SIDE VIEW

Sea mammal skeletons

SEA MAMMALS INCLUDE ANIMALS that spend their life in water, such as whales and dolphins, and those that live mostly in water but come ashore to breed, such as seals, sea lions, and walruses. All evolved from land-living mammals, and their skeletons show numerous adaptations to aquatic life. Seal forelimbs and hind limbs are modified to form flippers, with short arm and leg bones and long phalanges (finger and toe bones). Earless seals use their front flippers for steering and their hind flippers for propulsion. In contrast, fur seals and sea lions use their front flippers for propulsion and their hind flippers for steering. A seal's backbone is highly flexible, allowing rapid turning in water and caterpillar-like shuffling movements on land. The whale skeleton produces a streamlined, fishlike shape, with an elongated head, a short neck, and a long, tapering body with no hind limbs. The forelimbs, which are used for steering, have shortened arm bones and extra phalanges (finger bones) to increase rigidity. Muscles attached above and below the whale's long, flexible backbone contract alternately to move the tail flukes up and down

Lumbar vertebrae

Sacrum

Caudal vertebrae

Ilium

Ischium

Femur

Tibia

Fibula

Tarsals

Metatarsals

Lumbar vertebrae

Phalanges

SEAL

Caudal vertebrae

Transverse process

Chevron

Neural spine

KILLER WHALE

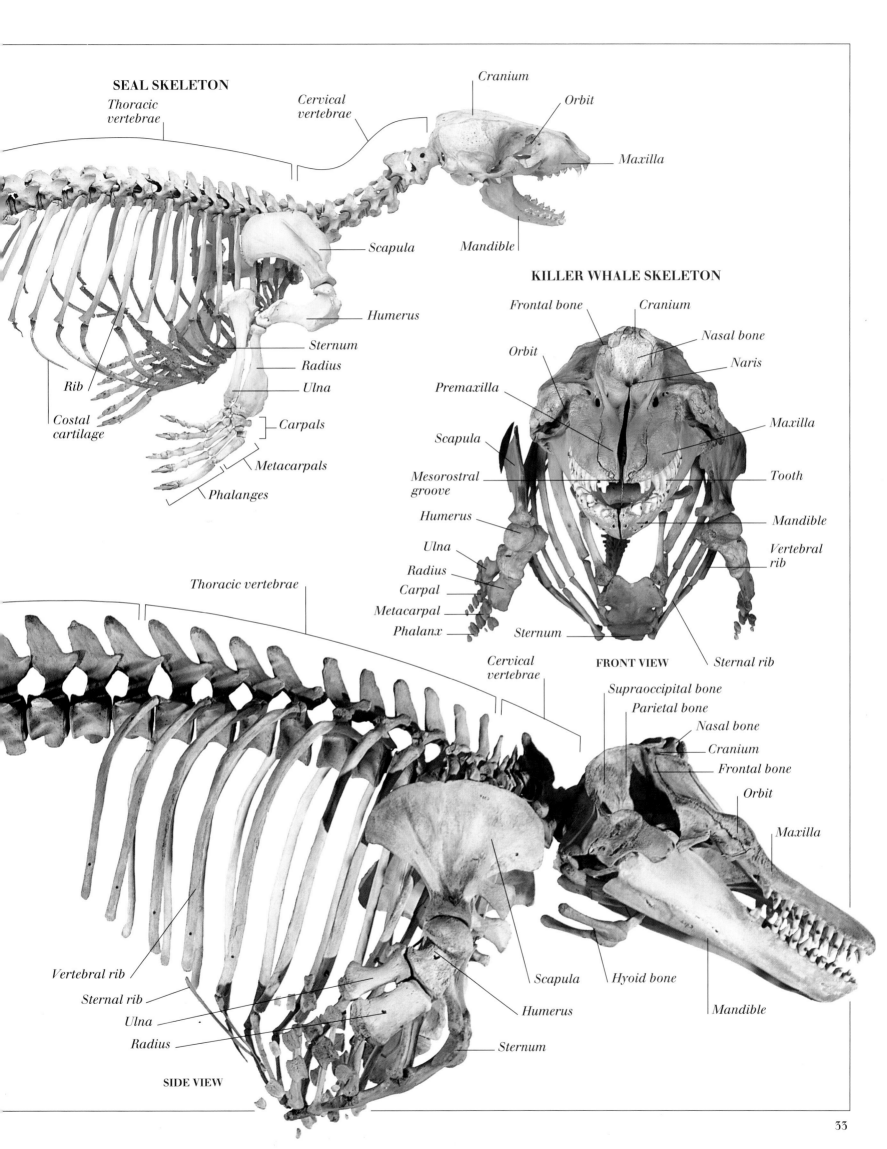

SEAL SKELETON

Thoracic vertebrae

Cervical vertebrae

Cranium

Orbit

Maxilla

Mandible

Scapula

Humerus

Sternum

Radius

Ulna

Rib

Carpals

Costal cartilage

Metacarpals

Phalanges

KILLER WHALE SKELETON

Frontal bone

Cranium

Orbit

Nasal bone

Naris

Premaxilla

Maxilla

Scapula

Mesorostral groove

Tooth

Humerus

Mandible

Ulna

Vertebral rib

Radius

Carpal

Metacarpal

Phalanx

Sternum

Sternal rib

Cervical vertebrae

FRONT VIEW

Thoracic vertebrae

Supraoccipital bone

Parietal bone

Nasal bone

Cranium

Frontal bone

Orbit

Maxilla

Scapula

Hyoid bone

Vertebral rib

Humerus

Mandible

Sternal rib

Ulna

Radius

Sternum

SIDE VIEW

33

Land mammal skeletons 1

LAND MAMMALS, unlike those that live in the sea, are not supported by the medium that surrounds them. Their entire weight is supported by the skeleton, in particular the strong vertebral column (backbone), and limbs that act as struts to hold the body off the ground. Mammals vary in the way the limbs support their body weight. In small, scampering mammals, such as squirrels and guinea pigs, the whole foot lies flat on the ground. Larger mammals typically raise the heel off the ground: cats and tigers walk on their toes, and horses walk on one hoofed digit. The elephant has pillarlike limb bones to support its weight. However, not all land mammals fit into this pattern. For example, the platypus has short, broad limbs, but is adapted more for swimming than walking, whereas the bat's forelimbs are adapted for flight. The kangaroo hops on its hind limbs and uses its tail for balance and support.

BAT SKELETON

BAT

- Skull
- Carpal
- Mandible
- Clavicle
- Sternum
- Radius
- Metacarpal
- Ulna
- Thoracic vertebra
- Femur
- Tarsal
- Metatarsal
- Phalanx
- Tibia
- Phalanx

PLATYPUS SKELETON

- Premaxilla
- Mandible
- Maxilla
- Cranium
- Atlas
- Orbit
- Axis
- Claw
- Phalanx
- Scapula
- Metacarpal
- Radius
- Carpal
- Ulna
- Humerus
- Rib
- Costal enlargement of rib
- Epipubic bone
- Sacrum
- Femur
- Ilium
- Ischium
- Fibula
- Phalanx
- Tibia
- Metatarsal
- Tarsal
- Patella

PLATYPUS

- Lumbar vertebra
- Sacrum
- Ilium
- Ischium
- Caudal vertebra
- Pubis
- Patella
- Femur
- Calcaneus
- Tibia
- Fibula
- Tarsal
- Metatarsal
- Phalanx
- Retractable claw

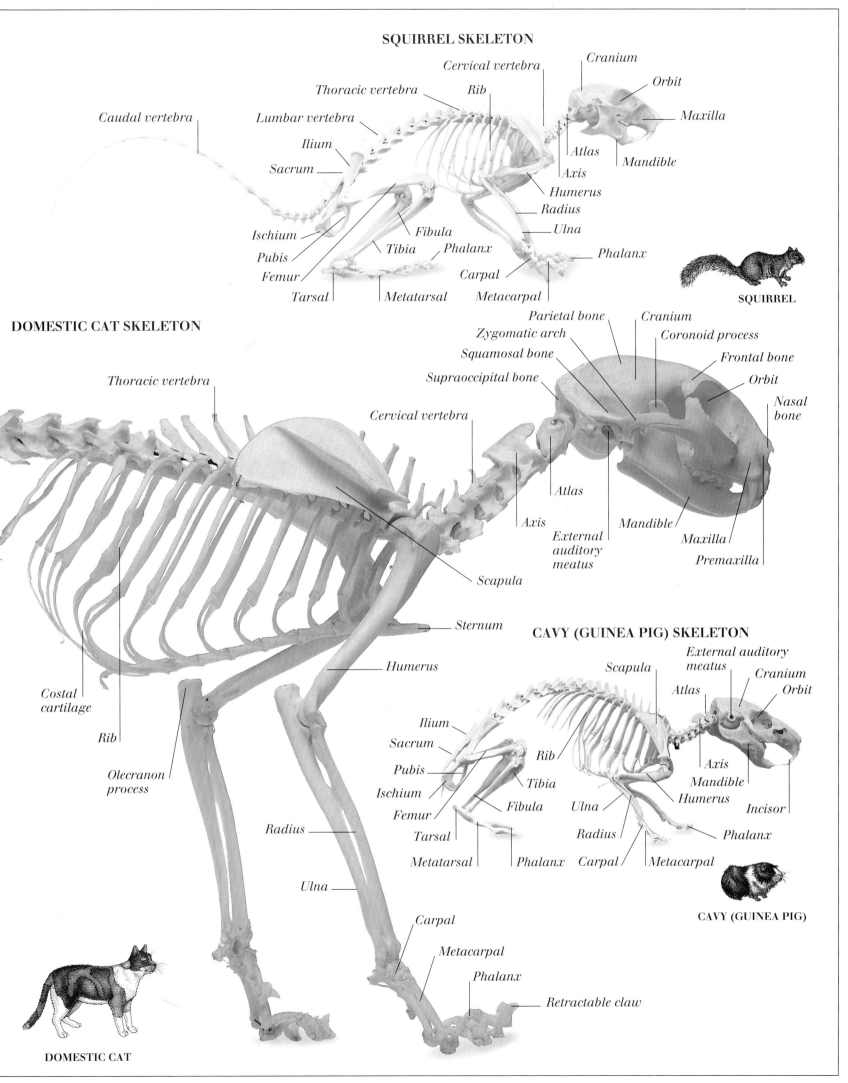

SQUIRREL SKELETON

Cranium
Cervical vertebra
Orbit
Thoracic vertebra
Rib
Maxilla
Caudal vertebra
Lumbar vertebra
Ilium
Atlas
Mandible
Sacrum
Axis
Humerus
Radius
Ulna
Ischium
Fibula
Pubis
Tibia
Phalanx
Phalanx
Femur
Carpal
Tarsal
Metatarsal
Metacarpal

SQUIRREL

DOMESTIC CAT SKELETON

Parietal bone
Cranium
Zygomatic arch
Coronoid process
Squamosal bone
Frontal bone
Supraoccipital bone
Orbit
Thoracic vertebra
Nasal bone
Cervical vertebra
Atlas
Axis
Mandible
External auditory meatus
Maxilla
Premaxilla
Scapula
Sternum

CAVY (GUINEA PIG) SKELETON

External auditory meatus
Scapula
Cranium
Atlas
Orbit
Ilium
Rib
Sacrum
Axis
Pubis
Mandible
Ischium
Tibia
Humerus
Femur
Fibula
Incisor
Tarsal
Ulna
Phalanx
Metatarsal
Phalanx
Radius
Carpal
Metacarpal
Humerus

CAVY (GUINEA PIG)

Costal cartilage
Rib
Olecranon process
Radius
Ulna
Carpal
Metacarpal
Phalanx
Retractable claw

DOMESTIC CAT

Land mammal skeletons 2

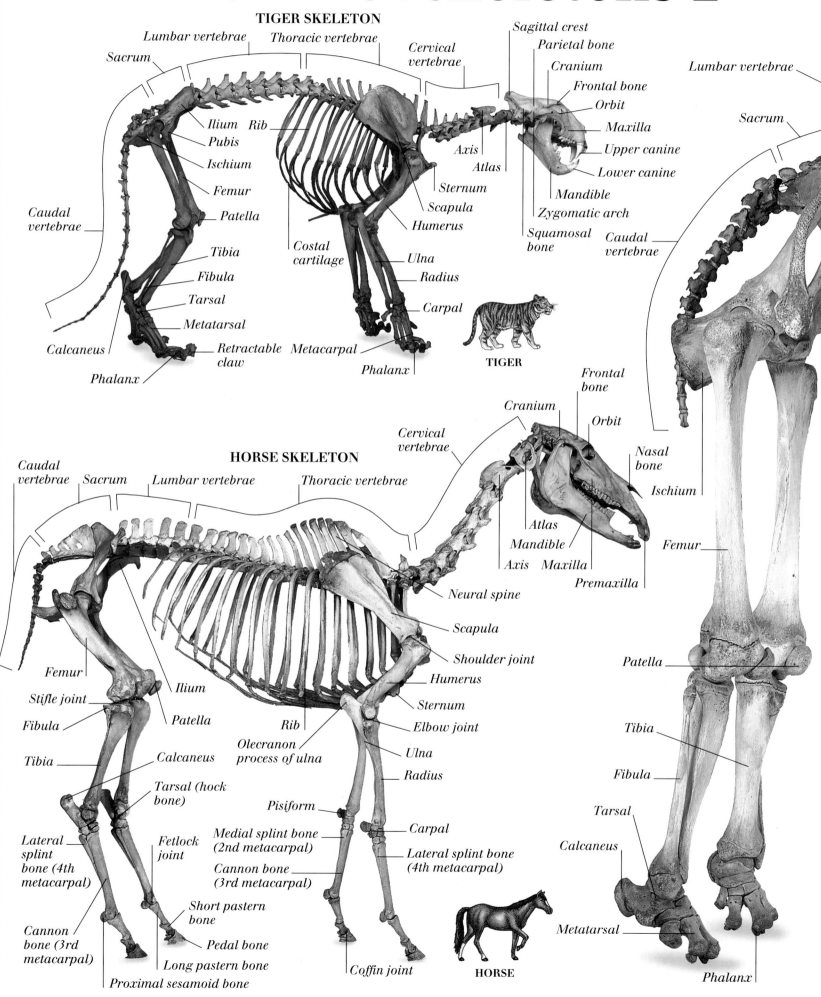

TIGER SKELETON

Lumbar vertebrae
Thoracic vertebrae
Cervical vertebrae
Sagittal crest
Parietal bone
Cranium
Frontal bone
Orbit
Sacrum
Ilium
Rib
Maxilla
Pubis
Upper canine
Axis
Lower canine
Ischium
Atlas
Mandible
Femur
Sternum
Zygomatic arch
Caudal vertebrae
Patella
Scapula
Humerus
Squamosal bone
Tibia
Costal cartilage
Fibula
Ulna
Tarsal
Radius
Metatarsal
Carpal
Calcaneus
Retractable claw
Metacarpal
Phalanx
Phalanx

TIGER

Lumbar vertebrae
Sacrum
Caudal vertebrae

Frontal bone
Cranium
Orbit
Cervical vertebrae
Nasal bone
Ischium
Atlas
Mandible
Maxilla
Axis
Premaxilla
Femur

HORSE SKELETON

Caudal vertebrae
Sacrum
Lumbar vertebrae
Thoracic vertebrae
Neural spine
Scapula
Shoulder joint
Humerus
Femur
Ilium
Sternum
Stifle joint
Patella
Rib
Elbow joint
Fibula
Olecranon process of ulna
Ulna
Tibia
Calcaneus
Radius
Tarsal (hock bone)
Patella
Pisiform
Lateral splint bone (4th metacarpal)
Fetlock joint
Medial splint bone (2nd metacarpal)
Carpal
Tibia
Cannon bone (3rd metacarpal)
Lateral splint bone (4th metacarpal)
Fibula
Cannon bone (3rd metacarpal)
Short pastern bone
Tarsal
Pedal bone
Calcaneus
Long pastern bone
Coffin joint
Metatarsal
Proximal sesamoid bone

HORSE

Phalanx

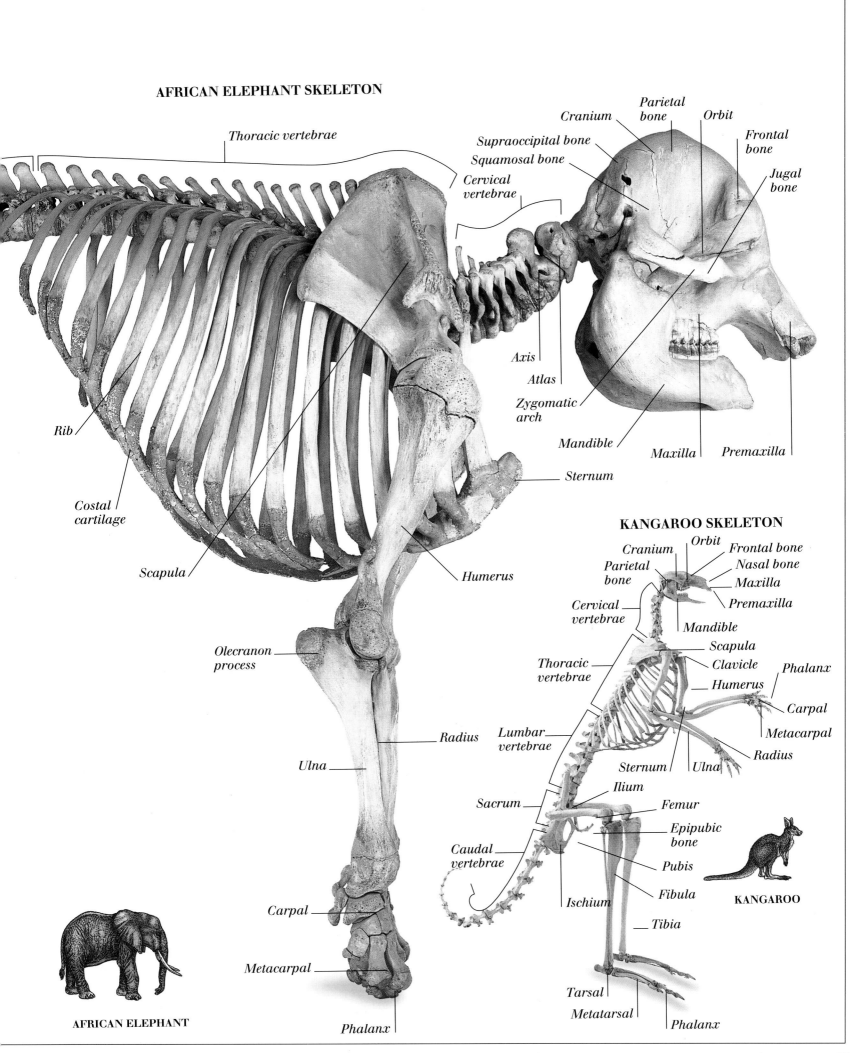

AFRICAN ELEPHANT SKELETON

Thoracic vertebrae

Cranium

Parietal bone

Orbit

Supraoccipital bone

Frontal bone

Squamosal bone

Cervical vertebrae

Jugal bone

Axis

Atlas

Zygomatic arch

Mandible

Maxilla

Premaxilla

Sternum

Rib

KANGAROO SKELETON

Cranium

Orbit

Frontal bone

Parietal bone

Nasal bone

Maxilla

Premaxilla

Cervical vertebrae

Mandible

Scapula

Clavicle

Phalanx

Humerus

Carpal

Metacarpal

Radius

Ulna

Sternum

Humerus

Costal cartilage

Scapula

Thoracic vertebrae

Lumbar vertebrae

Ilium

Femur

Epipubic bone

Sacrum

Olecranon process

Pubis

Caudal vertebrae

Fibula

Ischium

KANGAROO

Radius

Ulna

Tibia

Carpal

Tarsal

AFRICAN ELEPHANT

Metacarpal

Metatarsal

Phalanx

Phalanx

37

Early human relatives

THE DEVELOPMENT OF the modern human skeleton has involved changes associated with the shift from a quadrupedal (four-footed) stance to an upright, bipedal (two-footed) stance, and also with an enlarging cranium. Apelike *Proconsul africanus*, which lived 20 million years ago, had the long pelvis and arms typical of a quadrupedal stance. However, hominid fossil remains from 5 million years ago have strong leg bones, a broad pelvis, and an S-shaped backbone, suggesting a bipedal stance. These features can be seen in 3-million-year-old *Australopithecus afarensis* ("Lucy"), and also in later skeletons such as those of *Homo erectus* (Upright Man), *Homo neanderthalensis* (Neanderthal Man), and *Homo sapiens* (modern human). However, *Homo sapiens* has a larger brain than its ancestors, with a smaller face and jaw. All whole skeletons and external views shown here are reconstructions.

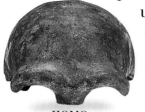

HOMO
NEANDERTHALENSIS
CRANIUM

AUSTRALOPITHECUS AFARENSIS ("LUCY")

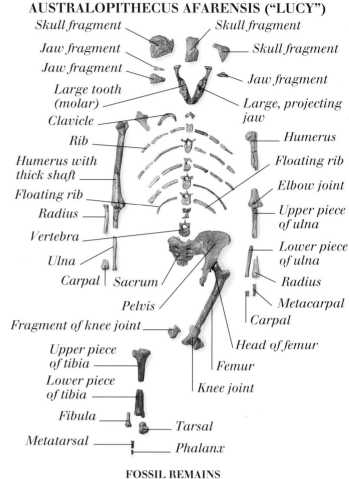

Skull fragment
Jaw fragment
Jaw fragment
Large tooth (molar)
Clavicle
Rib
Humerus with thick shaft
Floating rib
Radius
Vertebra
Ulna
Carpal
Sacrum
Pelvis
Fragment of knee joint
Upper piece of tibia
Lower piece of tibia
Fibula
Metatarsal

Skull fragment
Skull fragment
Jaw fragment
Large, projecting jaw
Humerus
Floating rib
Elbow joint
Upper piece of ulna
Lower piece of ulna
Radius
Metacarpal
Carpal
Head of femur
Femur
Knee joint
Tarsal
Phalanx

FOSSIL REMAINS

PROCONSUL AFRICANUS

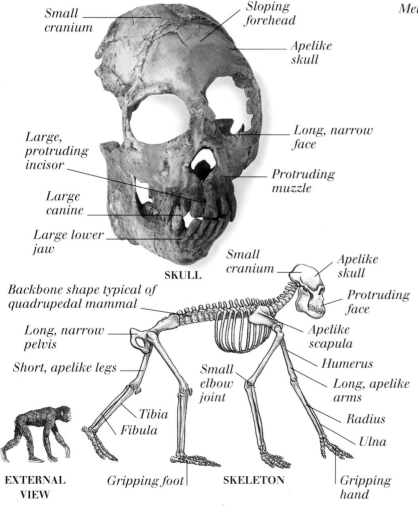

Small cranium
Sloping forehead
Apelike skull
Large, protruding incisor
Long, narrow face
Protruding muzzle
Large canine
Large lower jaw

SKULL

Backbone shape typical of quadrupedal mammal
Long, narrow pelvis
Short, apelike legs
Tibia
Fibula
Small cranium
Apelike skull
Protruding face
Apelike scapula
Humerus
Small elbow joint
Long, apelike arms
Radius
Ulna
Gripping hand
Gripping foot

EXTERNAL VIEW
SKELETON

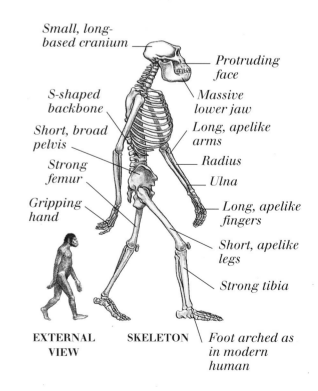

Small, long-based cranium
Protruding face
Massive lower jaw
S-shaped backbone
Short, broad pelvis
Long, apelike arms
Strong femur
Radius
Gripping hand
Ulna
Long, apelike fingers
Short, apelike legs
Strong tibia

EXTERNAL VIEW
SKELETON
Foot arched as in modern human

HOMO ERECTUS

Sloping forehead

Smaller cranium

Thick skull

Prominent supraorbital ridge

Sloping forehead

Wide-set eyes

Deep, flat cheekbone

Broad, flat nose

Wide face

SKULL

HOMO NEANDERTHALENSIS

Large, flat-topped cranium

Thinner skull

Prominent supraorbital ridge

Domed forehead

Close-set eyes

Wide-set eyes

Long face

Hard, strong teeth

Large mandible

No chin (mandibular protuberance)

SKULL

HOMO SAPIENS

Rounded cranium

Thin skull

Domed forehead

Hard, strong teeth

Small mandible

More prominent chin (mandibular protuberance)

SKULL

Small, long-based cranium

Slightly protruding face

Scapula

Rib

S-shaped backbone

Radius

Short, broad pelvis

Ulna

Femur

Long, thick tibia

Long legs

Long fibula

EXTERNAL VIEW

SKELETON

Prominent supraorbital ridge

Low, flat-topped, short-based cranium

Less prominent cheekbones

Scapula

Large mandible

Thick-shafted humerus

Rib

Large elbow joint

Radius

S-shaped backbone

Ulna

Short, broad pelvis

Long thumb

Gripping hand

Short, thick tibia

Thick, curved femur

Short fibula

Large ankle joint

EXTERNAL VIEW

SKELETON

Reduced supraorbital ridge

Domed forehead

Large, short-based cranium

Small mandible

Scapula

Flat face

Humerus

Rib

S-shaped backbone

Ulna

Radius

Short, broad pelvis

Opposable thumb

Long femur

Long tibia

Long fibula

EXTERNAL VIEW

SKELETON

Bone structure and function

LIVING BONE IS A HARD, constantly changing, self-repairing tissue that is supplied with blood vessels and nerves. It consists of bone cells and the intercellular matrix that lies between them. About 65 percent of this matrix consists of mineral salts, mainly calcium phosphate, which give bone its hardness; the other 35 percent consists mainly of collagen fibers, which provide flexibility. Bones have a thin outer coat of periosteum, containing osteoblasts (bone-forming cells) and osteoclasts (bone-destroying cells). Within the periosteum is a layer of compact bone consisting of concentric cylinders (lamellae) of matrix called osteons (Haversian systems), each of which acts as a weight-bearing pillar. Osteons are laid down around a central (Haversian) canal, which contains the blood vessels that supply osteocytes (mature bone cells) with nutrients and oxygen; adjacent Haversian canals are connected by Volkmann's canals. Osteocytes, found in lacunae (chambers) at the junctions of lamellae, maintain the bone matrix and communicate through dendrites (cell processes) that pass along tiny canals known as canaliculi. Spongy (cancellous) bone is situated within compact bone and consists of struts (trabeculae) that make it both light and strong. Red bone marrow, found in the spaces within cancellous bone, produces red and white blood cells.

MICROGRAPH OF LAMELLA FRAGMENT

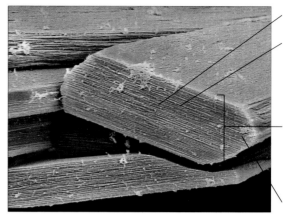

Bone matrix

Layers of collagen fibers and mineral salts

Lamella (layer of bone)

Crystallites aligned parallel to collagen fibers

MICROGRAPH OF SPONGY BONE

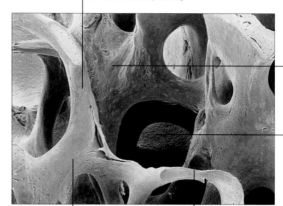

Trabecula (strut)

Trabecular plate

Marrow space

Bifurcation

Trabecular bar

MICROGRAPH OF OSTEON

Blood vessels, nerves, and lymphatic vessels in Haversian canal

Lacuna

Lamella

Osteon

Lacuna

STRUCTURAL FEATURES OF BONE

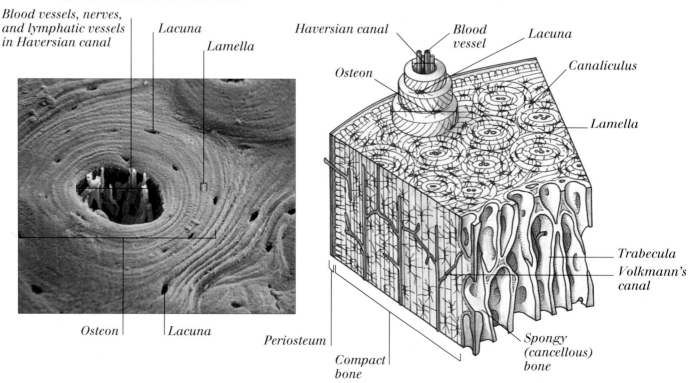

Haversian canal

Blood vessel

Lacuna

Osteon

Canaliculus

Lamella

Trabecula

Volkmann's canal

Periosteum

Spongy (cancellous) bone

Compact bone

MICROGRAPH OF OSTEOCYTE IN LACUNA

Canaliculus *Lacuna* *Bone matrix*

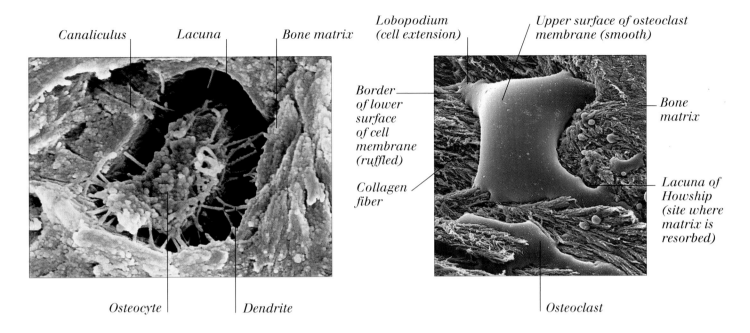

Osteocyte *Dendrite*

MICROGRAPH OF OSTEOCLAST

Lobopodium (cell extension) *Upper surface of osteoclast membrane (smooth)*

Border of lower surface of cell membrane (ruffled) *Bone matrix*

Collagen fiber *Lacuna of Howship (site where matrix is resorbed)*

Osteoclast

MICROGRAPH OF RED BONE MARROW

Lymphocyte *Monocyte* *Neutrophil*

Basophilic normoblast

Polychromatic normoblast

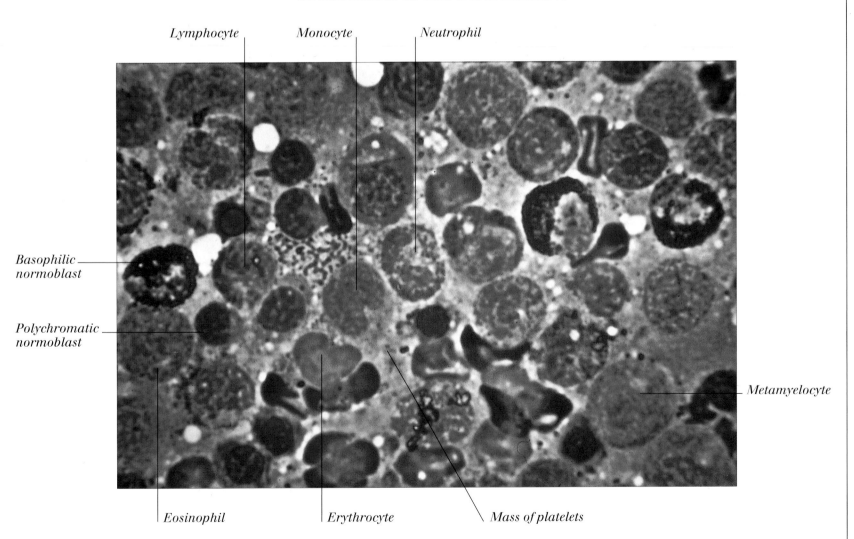

Metamyelocyte

Eosinophil *Erythrocyte* *Mass of platelets*

41

Joints

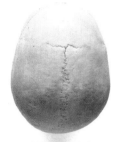

SUTURES OF SKULL

A JOINT IS A SITE where two or more bones meet. Joints have two main functions: to allow movement, and to maintain stability. Tough, inelastic ligaments prevent joint dislocation. There are three types of joints: immobile fibrous joints, such as the sutures between skull bones; slightly movable cartilaginous joints, such as those between vertebrae; and highly mobile synovial joints. Most body joints are synovial. To enable smooth movement, the ends of the bones of synovial joints are covered with glassy hyaline cartilage, and separated by a cavity filled with synovial fluid. Five main types of synovial joints are found in mammals: pivot joints permit rotation of one bone against or inside another; ball-and-socket joints allow movement in all directions; hinge joints allow bending and straightening only; saddle joints permit backward and forward, and side-to-side movements; and plane joints allow short, gliding movements.

HIP JOINT LIGAMENTS

ANATOMY OF HIP JOINT

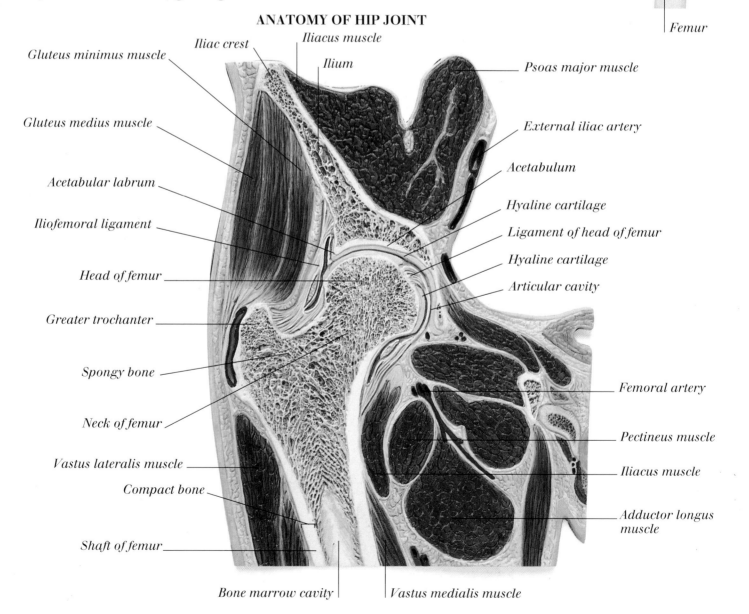

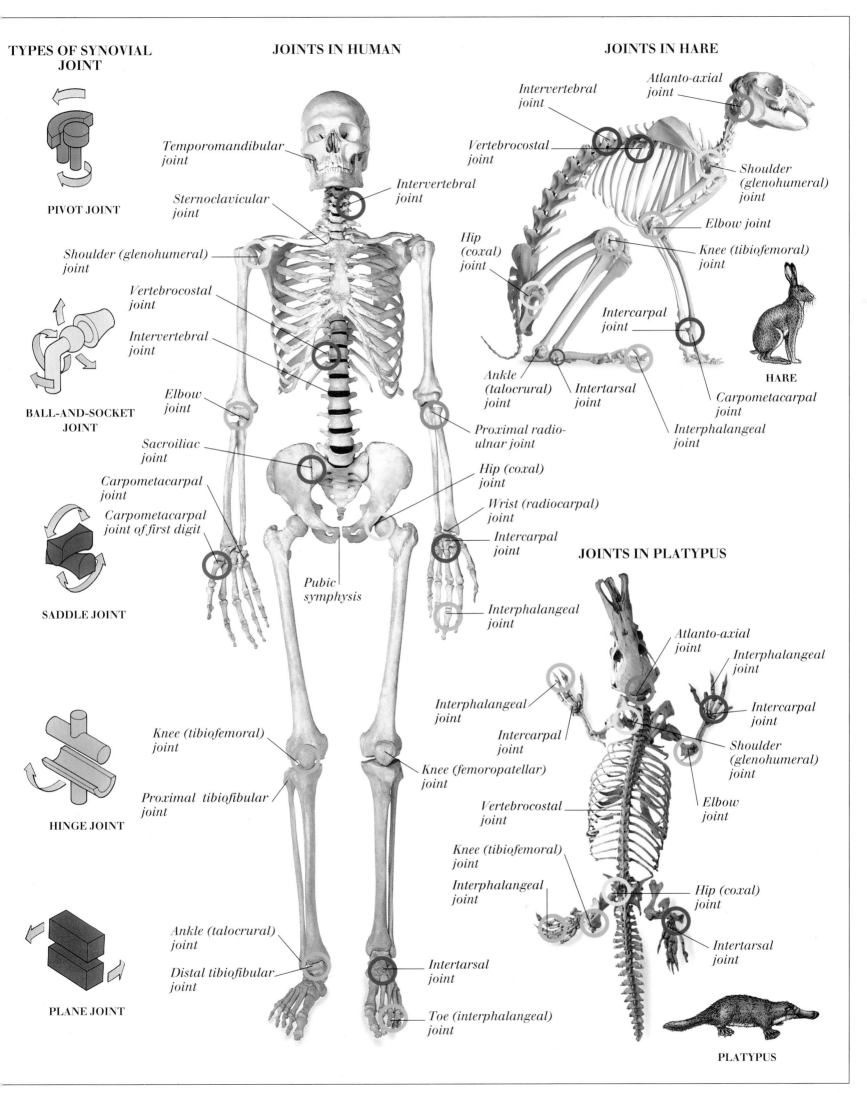

TYPES OF SYNOVIAL JOINT

PIVOT JOINT

BALL-AND-SOCKET JOINT

SADDLE JOINT

HINGE JOINT

PLANE JOINT

JOINTS IN HUMAN

Temporomandibular joint

Sternoclavicular joint

Intervertebral joint

Shoulder (glenohumeral) joint

Vertebrocostal joint

Intervertebral joint

Elbow joint

Sacroiliac joint

Carpometacarpal joint

Carpometacarpal joint of first digit

Proximal radio-ulnar joint

Hip (coxal) joint

Wrist (radiocarpal) joint

Intercarpal joint

Pubic symphysis

Interphalangeal joint

Knee (tibiofemoral) joint

Knee (femoropatellar) joint

Proximal tibiofibular joint

Ankle (talocrural) joint

Distal tibiofibular joint

Intertarsal joint

Toe (interphalangeal) joint

JOINTS IN HARE

Intervertebral joint

Atlanto-axial joint

Vertebrocostal joint

Shoulder (glenohumeral) joint

Elbow joint

Hip (coxal) joint

Knee (tibiofemoral) joint

Intercarpal joint

Ankle (talocrural) joint

Intertarsal joint

Carpometacarpal joint

Interphalangeal joint

HARE

JOINTS IN PLATYPUS

Atlanto-axial joint

Interphalangeal joint

Intercarpal joint

Shoulder (glenohumeral) joint

Elbow joint

Interphalangeal joint

Intercarpal joint

Vertebrocostal joint

Knee (tibiofemoral) joint

Interphalangeal joint

Hip (coxal) joint

Intertarsal joint

PLATYPUS

Human skulls

THE BONES OF THE HUMAN SKULL serve several functions. Cranial bones surround and protect the brain. Facial bones provide attachment points for facial muscles, openings for eating and breathing, cavities for the sensory organs, and anchorage for the teeth. With the exception of the mandible (lower jaw) and the ear ossicles, the skull bones are knitted together by immovable joints called sutures. Blood vessels, nerves, and the spinal cord cross the skull through foramina (holes). The bone structure of early human skulls differs greatly from that of modern humans. The 200,000-year-old skull of *Homo heidelbergensis* (originally called "Rhodesian Man") has no forehead, prominent supraorbital (brow) ridges, and a large upper jaw. The 38,000-year-old skull from La Ferrassie is an example of *Homo neanderthalensis* ("Neanderthal Man"), who lived 100,000 to 35,000 years ago, immediately preceding *Homo sapiens* (modern human) in Europe. *Homo neanderthalensis* had heavy supraorbital ridges and a sharply sloping forehead. *Homo sapiens* has a more domed forehead, a flatter face, and a smaller jaw.

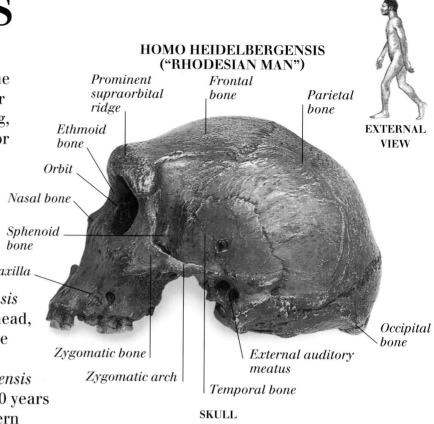

HOMO HEIDELBERGENSIS ("RHODESIAN MAN")

Prominent supraorbital ridge

Frontal bone

Parietal bone

EXTERNAL VIEW

Ethmoid bone

Orbit

Nasal bone

Sphenoid bone

Maxilla

Zygomatic bone

Zygomatic arch

Temporal bone

External auditory meatus

Occipital bone

SKULL

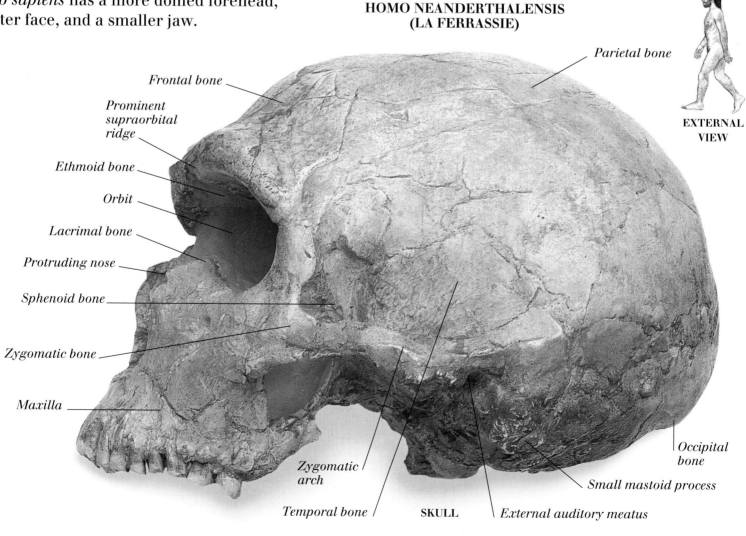

HOMO NEANDERTHALENSIS (LA FERRASSIE)

Parietal bone

EXTERNAL VIEW

Frontal bone

Prominent supraorbital ridge

Ethmoid bone

Orbit

Lacrimal bone

Protruding nose

Sphenoid bone

Zygomatic bone

Maxilla

Zygomatic arch

Temporal bone

SKULL

External auditory meatus

Small mastoid process

Occipital bone

HOMO SAPIENS SKULL

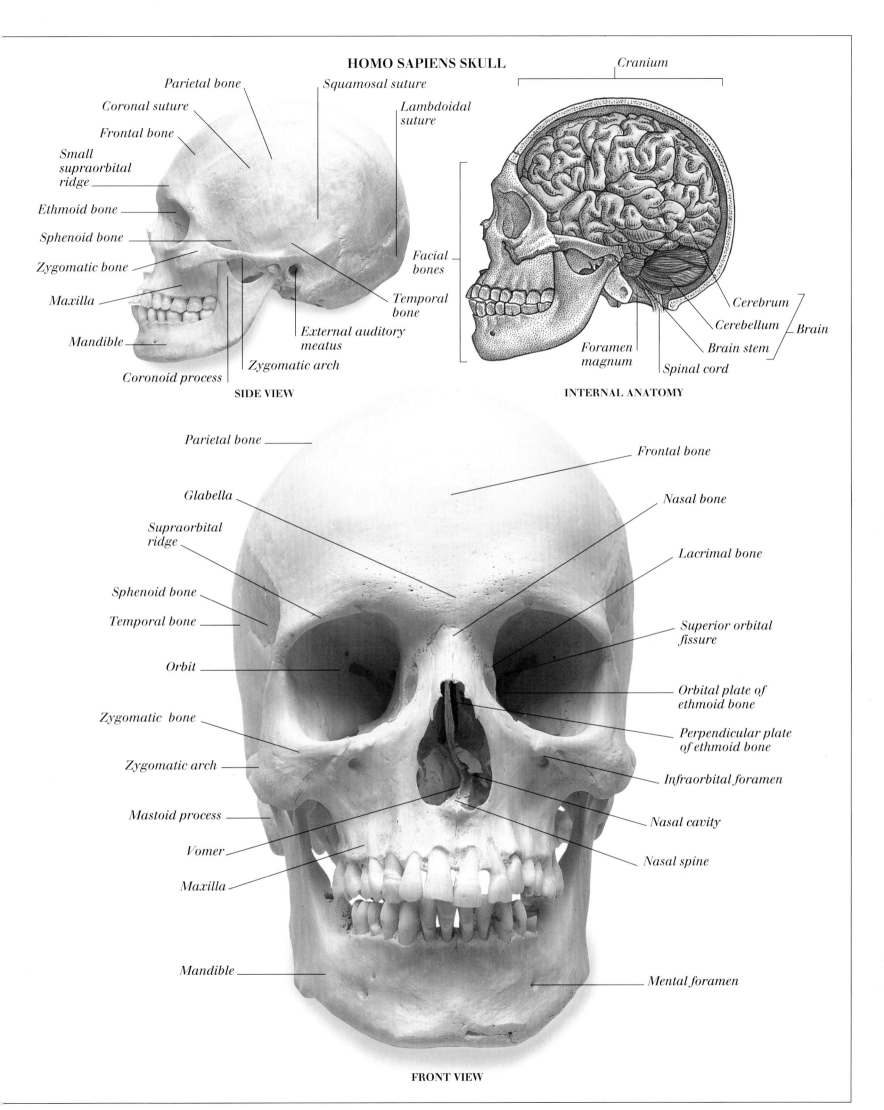

SIDE VIEW

Parietal bone

Coronal suture

Frontal bone

Small supraorbital ridge

Ethmoid bone

Sphenoid bone

Zygomatic bone

Maxilla

Mandible

Coronoid process

Zygomatic arch

Squamosal suture

Lambdoidal suture

Facial bones

Temporal bone

External auditory meatus

INTERNAL ANATOMY

Cranium

Cerebrum

Cerebellum

Brain stem

Brain

Foramen magnum

Spinal cord

FRONT VIEW

Parietal bone

Glabella

Supraorbital ridge

Sphenoid bone

Temporal bone

Orbit

Zygomatic bone

Zygomatic arch

Mastoid process

Vomer

Maxilla

Mandible

Frontal bone

Nasal bone

Lacrimal bone

Superior orbital fissure

Orbital plate of ethmoid bone

Perpendicular plate of ethmoid bone

Infraorbital foramen

Nasal cavity

Nasal spine

Mental foramen

Animal skulls

ALL VERTEBRATES HAVE A skull made of fused bones and a movable mandible (lower jaw). The function of the skull is to house and protect the brain and sensory organs, and to allow eating and breathing. Each species of animal has a skull shape adapted to its particular lifestyle. Typically, birds, such as vultures, have lightweight skulls that permit flight; carnivores (meat eaters), such as lions and crocodiles, have powerful jaws with sharp teeth; the toothless anteater has a long snout that enables it to probe into ant nests for food; and herbivores (plant eaters), such as the goat, have a loose-fitting lower jaw that permits side-to-side movement for grinding food. The two main muscles involved in biting and chewing are the temporalis and the masseter. In carnivores, both these muscles move the lower jaw up and down with a scissorlike action. In herbivores, the temporalis is relatively weak and the masseter provides the force needed to grind tough vegetation.

KING VULTURE SKULL

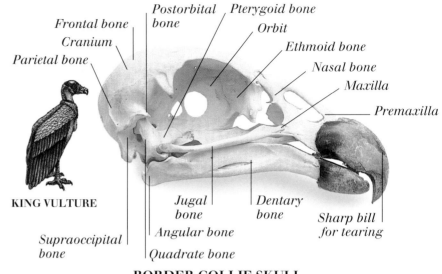

Frontal bone
Cranium
Parietal bone
Postorbital bone
Pterygoid bone
Orbit
Ethmoid bone
Nasal bone
Maxilla
Premaxilla
Jugal bone
Dentary bone
Sharp bill for tearing
Supraoccipital bone
Angular bone
Quadrate bone
KING VULTURE

BORDER COLLIE SKULL

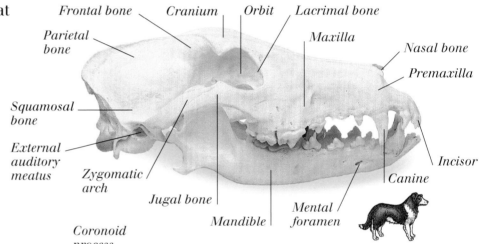

Frontal bone
Cranium
Orbit
Lacrimal bone
Parietal bone
Maxilla
Nasal bone
Premaxilla
Squamosal bone
External auditory meatus
Zygomatic arch
Jugal bone
Mandible
Mental foramen
Incisor
Canine
BORDER COLLIE

LION SKULL

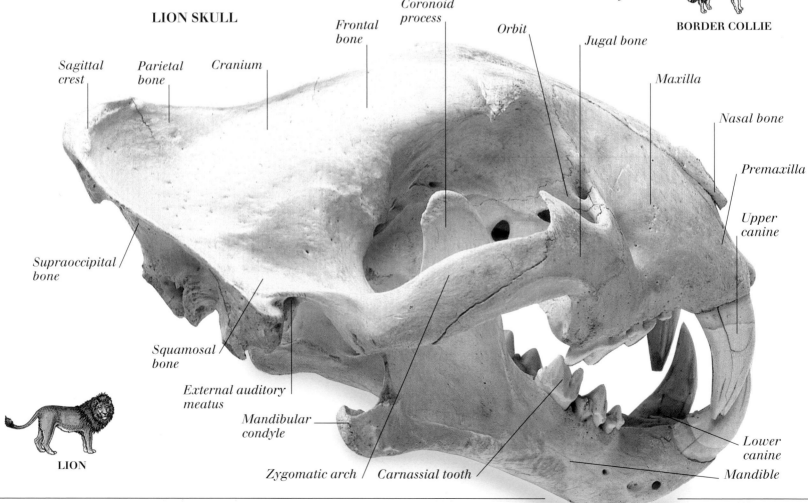

Sagittal crest
Parietal bone
Cranium
Frontal bone
Coronoid process
Orbit
Jugal bone
Maxilla
Nasal bone
Premaxilla
Upper canine
Supraoccipital bone
Squamosal bone
External auditory meatus
Mandibular condyle
Zygomatic arch
Carnassial tooth
Lower canine
Mandible
LION

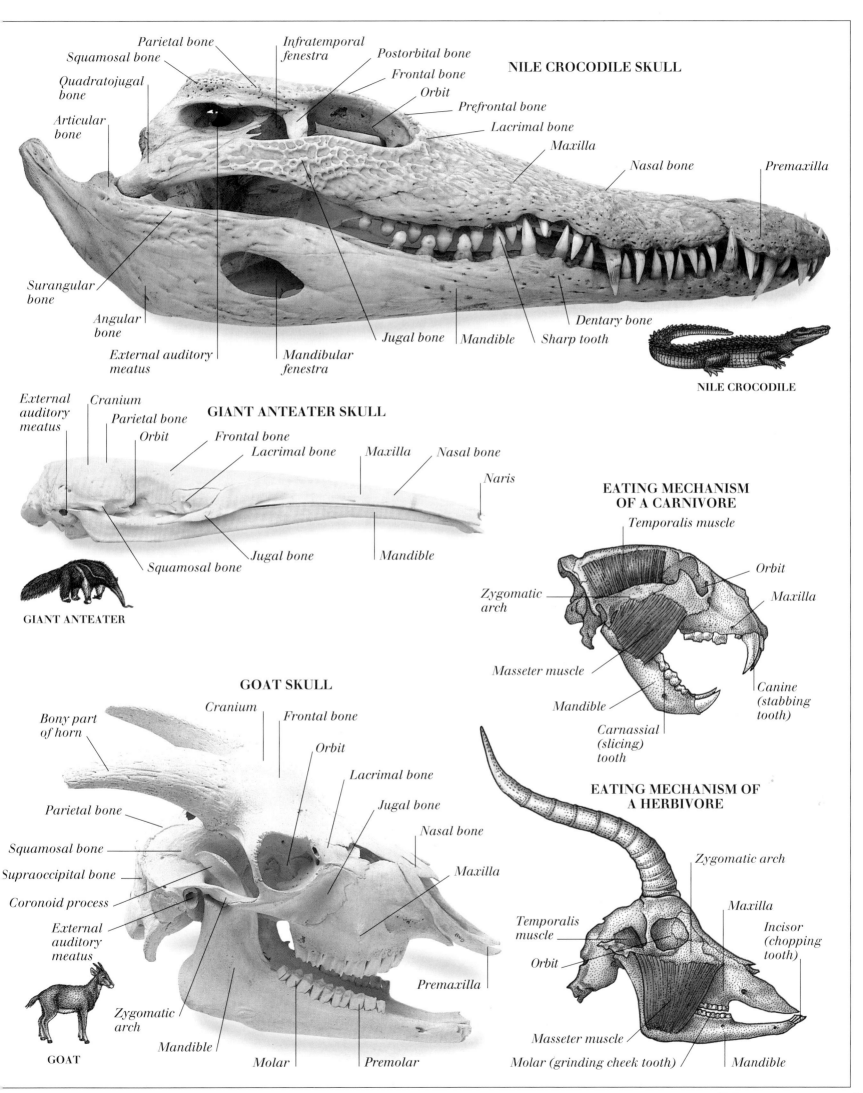

Parietal bone

Squamosal bone

Quadratojugal bone

Articular bone

Infratemporal fenestra

Postorbital bone

Frontal bone

Orbit

Prefrontal bone

Lacrimal bone

Maxilla

Nasal bone

Premaxilla

NILE CROCODILE SKULL

Surangular bone

Angular bone

External auditory meatus

Mandibular fenestra

Jugal bone

Mandible

Sharp tooth

Dentary bone

NILE CROCODILE

External auditory meatus

Cranium

Parietal bone

Orbit

Frontal bone

Lacrimal bone

Maxilla

Nasal bone

Naris

GIANT ANTEATER SKULL

Squamosal bone

Jugal bone

Mandible

GIANT ANTEATER

EATING MECHANISM OF A CARNIVORE

Temporalis muscle

Orbit

Maxilla

Zygomatic arch

Masseter muscle

Mandible

Canine (stabbing tooth)

Carnassial (slicing) tooth

GOAT SKULL

Cranium

Frontal bone

Bony part of horn

Orbit

Lacrimal bone

Jugal bone

Parietal bone

Nasal bone

Squamosal bone

Maxilla

Supraoccipital bone

Coronoid process

External auditory meatus

Premaxilla

Zygomatic arch

Mandible

Molar

Premolar

GOAT

EATING MECHANISM OF A HERBIVORE

Zygomatic arch

Maxilla

Incisor (chopping tooth)

Temporalis muscle

Orbit

Masseter muscle

Molar (grinding cheek tooth)

Mandible

Backbone

ALL VERTEBRATES HAVE A BACKBONE (vertebral column), which acts like a girder carrying the weight of the organs of the body. The backbone consists of a row of vertebrae separated by cartilaginous intervertebral disks that give limited flexibility. These vertebrae also form a protective tunnel around the spinal cord, while the neural spine and transverse processes of the vertebrae provide attachment points for muscles and ligaments. There are five types of vertebrae: cervical (neck), thoracic (chest), lumbar (abdominal), sacral (anchoring the backbone to the pelvis), and caudal (tail). Unlike most other vertebrates, birds have inflexible backbones—although the neck is flexible—to provide stability in flight. Most mammal backbones (such as the hare's) curve upward to help resist the downward pull of body weight, and vertebrae increase in size toward the lumbar end where stress is greatest. The human backbone is adapted to supporting the body in an upright position: it has an S-shaped curve that serves to position the body directly over the legs and feet.

ANATOMY OF HUMAN SPINAL COLUMN

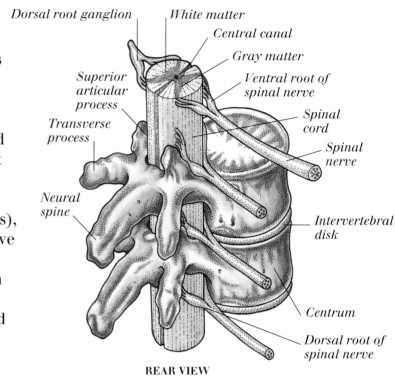

Dorsal root ganglion
White matter
Central canal
Gray matter
Superior articular process
Ventral root of spinal nerve
Transverse process
Spinal cord
Spinal nerve
Neural spine
Intervertebral disk
Centrum
Dorsal root of spinal nerve

REAR VIEW

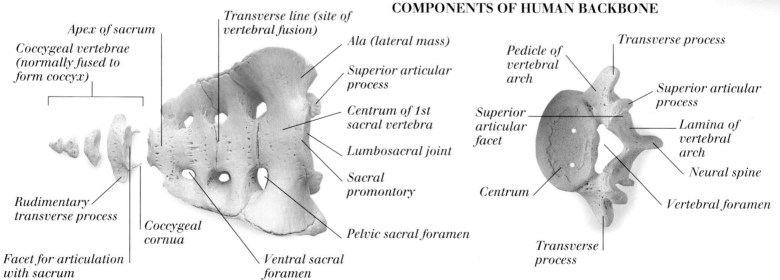

Lumbar vertebrae

Sacrum

Coccyx

Inferior articular process

Superior articular process

Centrum

COMPONENTS OF HUMAN BACKBONE

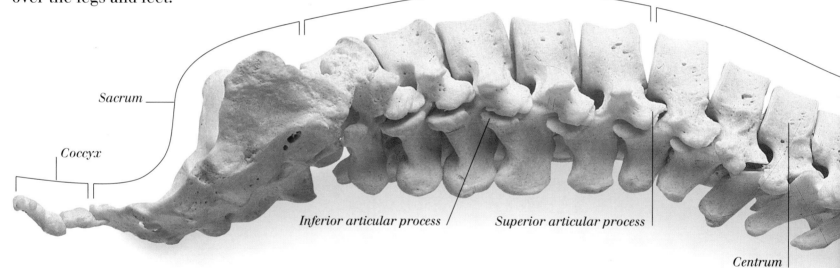

Apex of sacrum

Coccygeal vertebrae (normally fused to form coccyx)

Transverse line (site of vertebral fusion)

Ala (lateral mass)

Superior articular process

Centrum of 1st sacral vertebra

Lumbosacral joint

Sacral promontory

Pelvic sacral foramen

Rudimentary transverse process

Coccygeal cornua

Ventral sacral foramen

Facet for articulation with sacrum

Pedicle of vertebral arch

Transverse process

Superior articular process

Superior articular facet

Lamina of vertebral arch

Neural spine

Vertebral foramen

Centrum

Transverse process

FRONT VIEW OF SACRUM AND COCCYGEAL VERTEBRAE

TOP VIEW OF LUMBAR VERTEBRA

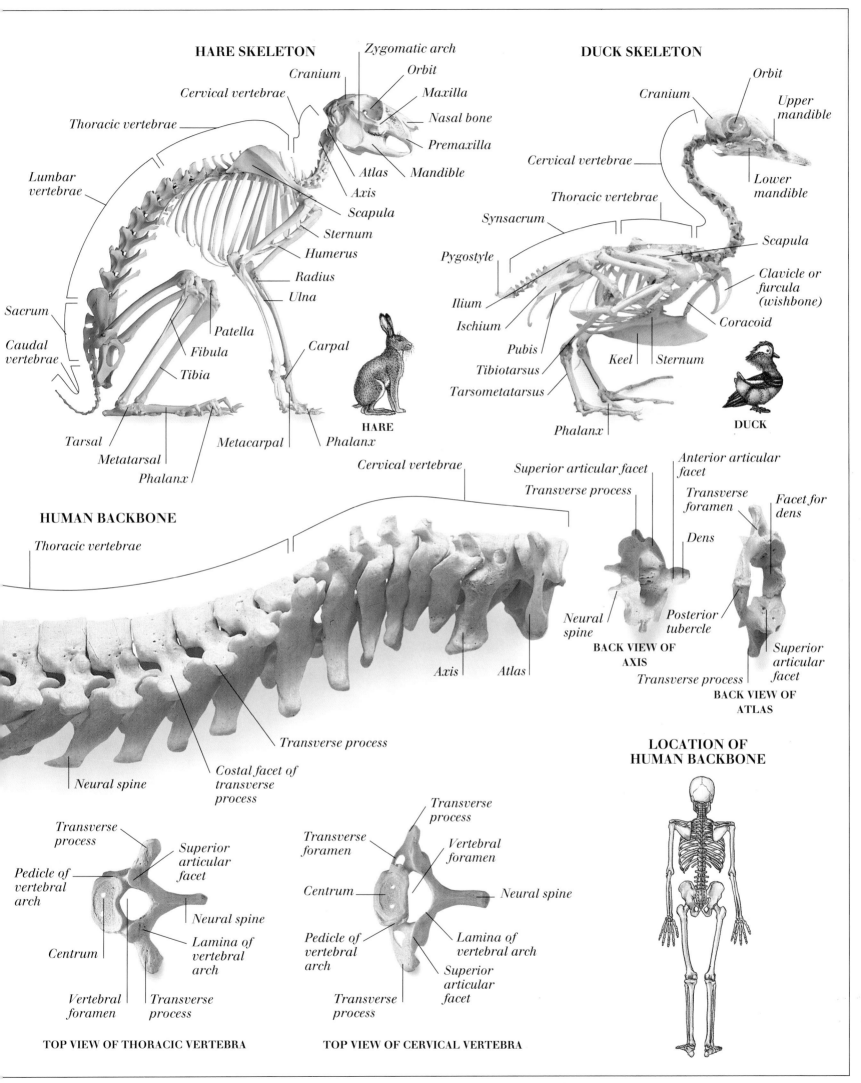

HARE SKELETON

Zygomatic arch
Cranium
Orbit
Maxilla
Nasal bone
Premaxilla
Cervical vertebrae
Thoracic vertebrae
Atlas
Mandible
Axis
Scapula
Lumbar vertebrae
Sternum
Humerus
Radius
Ulna
Sacrum
Caudal vertebrae
Patella
Fibula
Carpal
Tibia
Tarsal
Metatarsal
Phalanx
Metacarpal
Phalanx

HARE

DUCK SKELETON

Orbit
Cranium
Upper mandible
Cervical vertebrae
Lower mandible
Thoracic vertebrae
Synsacrum
Scapula
Pygostyle
Clavicle or furcula (wishbone)
Ilium
Coracoid
Ischium
Pubis
Tibiotarsus
Keel
Sternum
Tarsometatarsus
Phalanx

DUCK

HUMAN BACKBONE

Cervical vertebrae
Superior articular facet
Transverse process
Anterior articular facet
Transverse foramen
Facet for dens
Thoracic vertebrae
Dens
Neural spine
Posterior tubercle
Axis
Atlas
Transverse process

BACK VIEW OF AXIS

Superior articular facet

Transverse process

BACK VIEW OF ATLAS

Transverse process
Costal facet of transverse process
Neural spine

LOCATION OF HUMAN BACKBONE

Transverse process
Superior articular facet
Pedicle of vertebral arch
Neural spine
Centrum
Lamina of vertebral arch
Vertebral foramen
Transverse process

TOP VIEW OF THORACIC VERTEBRA

Transverse process
Transverse foramen
Vertebral foramen
Centrum
Neural spine
Pedicle of vertebral arch
Lamina of vertebral arch
Superior articular facet
Transverse process

TOP VIEW OF CERVICAL VERTEBRA

Ribcage

RIBS ARE CURVED, FLATTENED BONES found in all vertebrates. In land vertebrates, the ribs typically articulate with the thoracic vertebrae at one end and with the sternum (breastbone) at the other to form the ribcage. The ribcage protects the heart and lungs and is also flexible, allowing the lungs to inflate and deflate during breathing. Limbless vertebrates, such as snakes, have a tubular ribcage that supports the body and plays a part in locomotion. Humans have twelve pairs of ribs. Ribs 1–7, the true ribs, are attached to the sternum by costal cartilage. Ribs 8–12 are called the false ribs: ribs 8–10 are connected to one another by costal cartilage; ribs 11 and 12, the floating ribs, are connected only to the vertebral column. Breathing involves the action of the intercostal muscles (muscles between the ribs), and the diaphragm (the muscle sheet that separates the chest from the abdomen). When a person inhales (breathes in), the external intercostal muscles contract, moving the ribcage upward and outward, and the diaphragm contracts and flattens, drawing air into the lungs. When the person exhales (breathes out), the process is reversed, pushing air out of the lungs.

COBRA SKELETON

Cranium
Maxilla
Mandible
Vertebra
Rib
Articulation between rib and vertebra
Caudal vertebra

COBRA

CHILLINGHAM BULL SKELETON

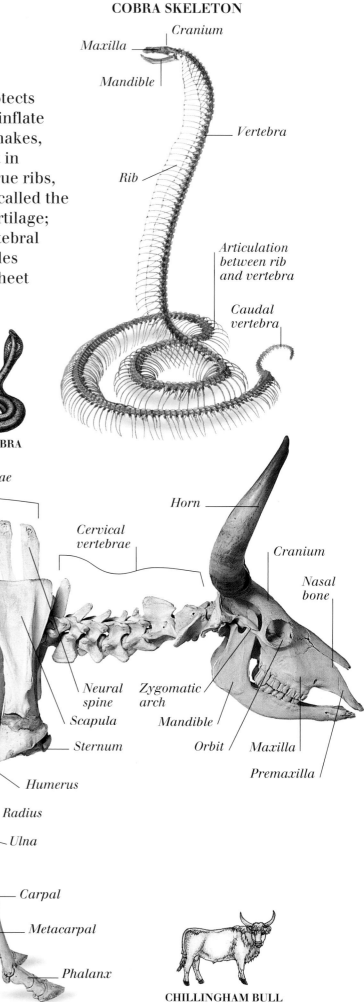

Thoracic vertebrae
Lumbar vertebrae
Sacrum
Caudal vertebrae
Cervical vertebrae
Horn
Cranium
Nasal bone
Ilium
Pubis
Ischium
Neural spine
Scapula
Zygomatic arch
Mandible
Orbit
Maxilla
Premaxilla
Femur
Patella
Costal cartilage
Sternum
Humerus
Rib
Radius
Tibia
Olecranon process
Ulna
Calcaneus
Tarsal
Carpal
Metatarsal
Metacarpal
Phalanx
Phalanx

CHILLINGHAM BULL

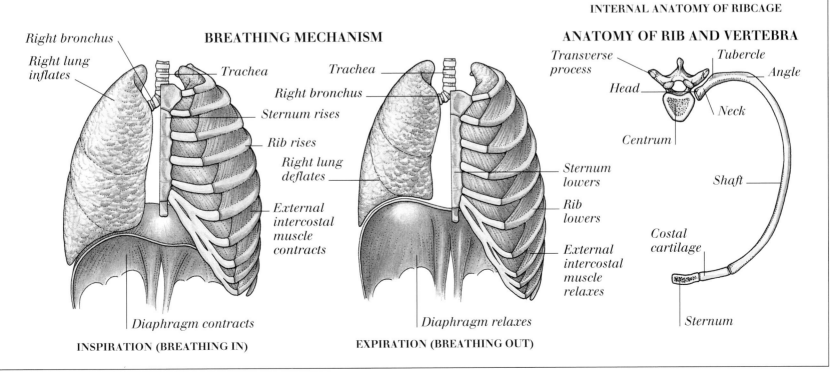

HUMAN RIBCAGE

Sternum
Jugular notch
Sternoclavicular joint
Clavicle
Scapula
Costal cartilage
Intercostal space
Shaft of rib
Thoracic vertebra
Intervertebral disk
11th rib
12th rib
Floating ribs
Lumbar vertebra
10th rib
1st rib
2nd rib
3rd rib
4th rib
5th rib
6th rib
7th rib
8th rib
9th rib

LOCATION OF RIBCAGE

INTERNAL ANATOMY OF RIBCAGE

Rib
Right lung
Left lung
Sternum
Heart located behind lungs
Costal cartilage
Liver
Stomach
Kidney
Ureter

BREATHING MECHANISM

Right bronchus
Right lung inflates
Trachea
Right lung deflates
Sternum rises
Rib rises
External intercostal muscle contracts
Diaphragm contracts

INSPIRATION (BREATHING IN)

Trachea
Right bronchus
Sternum lowers
Rib lowers
External intercostal muscle relaxes
Diaphragm relaxes

EXPIRATION (BREATHING OUT)

ANATOMY OF RIB AND VERTEBRA

Transverse process
Tubercle
Angle
Head
Neck
Centrum
Shaft
Costal cartilage
Sternum

Pelvis

THE PELVIS CONSISTS OF TWO COXAE (known as the pelvic girdle), the sacrum, and the coccyx. Together, these bones connect the hind limbs to the backbone, transmit the force from the hind limbs to the rest of the body, and support and protect the organs of the lower abdomen. Each coxa is formed by the fusion of three bones: the ilium, ischium, and pubis. The coxae are joined at a cartilaginous joint known as the pubic symphysis. The joints between the coxae and the sacrum are called the sacroiliac joints. Four-legged animals, such as dogs and cattle, typically have a horizontally aligned, elongated pelvis. Chimpanzees, with their semiupright posture, have an elongated, slightly tilted pelvis. In humans, who are fully upright, the pelvis is rounded and nearly vertical, so that the body is balanced directly over the feet.

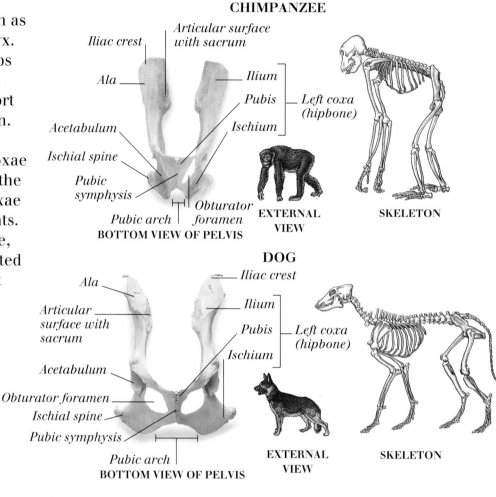

CHIMPANZEE

Iliac crest
Articular surface with sacrum
Ala
Ilium
Pubis
Left coxa (hipbone)
Ischium
Acetabulum
Ischial spine
Pubic symphysis
Obturator foramen
Pubic arch
BOTTOM VIEW OF PELVIS
EXTERNAL VIEW
SKELETON

DOG

Ala
Iliac crest
Articular surface with sacrum
Ilium
Pubis
Left coxa (hipbone)
Ischium
Acetabulum
Obturator foramen
Ischial spine
Pubic symphysis
Pubic arch
BOTTOM VIEW OF PELVIS
EXTERNAL VIEW
SKELETON

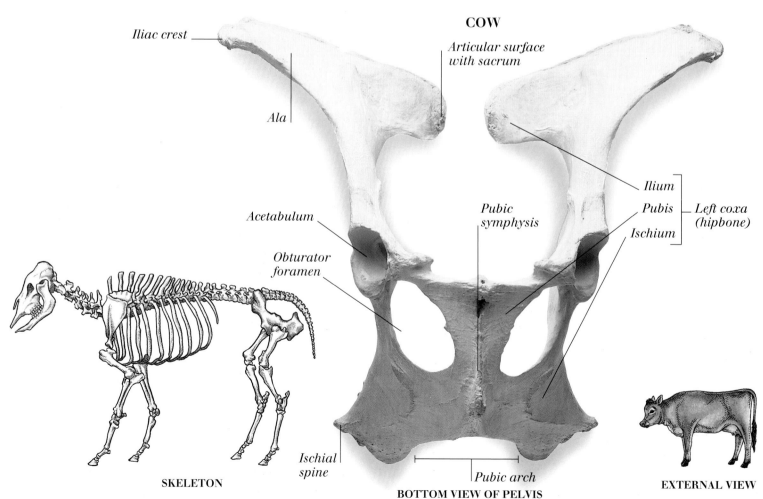

COW

Iliac crest
Articular surface with sacrum
Ala
Ilium
Pubis
Left coxa (hipbone)
Ischium
Acetabulum
Pubic symphysis
Obturator foramen
Ischial spine
Pubic arch
SKELETON
BOTTOM VIEW OF PELVIS
EXTERNAL VIEW

INTERNAL ANATOMY OF HUMAN PELVIS

LOCATION OF PELVIS

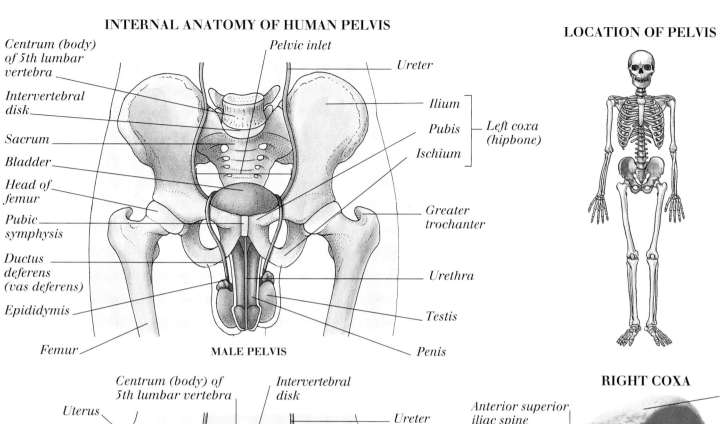

Centrum (body) of 5th lumbar vertebra

Intervertebral disk

Sacrum

Bladder

Head of femur

Pubic symphysis

Ductus deferens (vas deferens)

Epididymis

Femur

Pelvic inlet

Ureter

Ilium

Pubis — Left coxa (hipbone)

Ischium

Greater trochanter

Urethra

Testis

Penis

MALE PELVIS

Centrum (body) of 5th lumbar vertebra

Intervertebral disk

Uterus

Fimbriae

Ovary

Fallopian tube

Bladder

Head of femur

Pubic symphysis

Femur

Ureter

Sacrum

Ilium

Pubis — Left coxa

Ischium

Greater trochanter

Urethra

Vagina

FEMALE PELVIS

RIGHT COXA

Anterior superior iliac spine

Anterior inferior iliac spine

Acetabulum

Pubic tubercle

Pubis

Obturator foramen

Iliac crest

Ala of ilium

Ilium

Posterior superior iliac spine

Greater sciatic notch

Ischium

Ischial tuberosity

SIDE VIEW

COMPARISON OF MALE AND FEMALE PELVISES

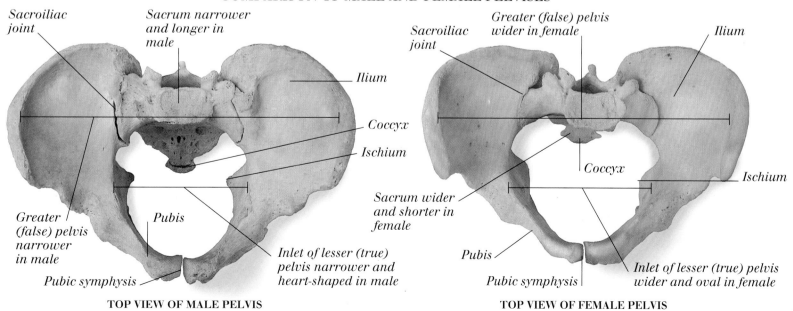

Sacroiliac joint

Sacrum narrower and longer in male

Ilium

Coccyx

Ischium

Greater (false) pelvis narrower in male

Pubis

Pubic symphysis

Inlet of lesser (true) pelvis narrower and heart-shaped in male

TOP VIEW OF MALE PELVIS

Sacroiliac joint

Greater (false) pelvis wider in female

Ilium

Coccyx

Sacrum wider and shorter in female

Ischium

Pubis

Pubic symphysis

Inlet of lesser (true) pelvis wider and oval in female

TOP VIEW OF FEMALE PELVIS

Forelimbs

THE FORELIMBS OF TETRAPODS (four-limbed vertebrates) are typically used for support, movement, and varying degrees of manipulation. They originated from an ancestral pentadactyl (five-fingered) forelimb. This would have consisted of a humerus (upper arm bone); an ulna and a radius (lower arm bones); ten carpals (wrist bones); five metacarpals (palm bones); and five sets of phalanges (finger bones). During evolution, the number, shape, and size of the forelimb bones changed to adapt vertebrates to particular lifestyles. For example, the short, strong forelimbs of the armadillo are adapted for digging; the arm and finger bones of the sea lion form a broad flipper for swimming; the gibbon's long arm bones and elongated, gripping fingers provide a secure hold on branches; and in flying vertebrates, such as the rock dove and bat, the forelimbs have become wings. Some fast-moving mammals— for example, horses and ponies—stand on a hoofed third digit; this is an adaptation for speed. The human forelimb is adapted mainly for intricate manipulation rather than support or locomotion.

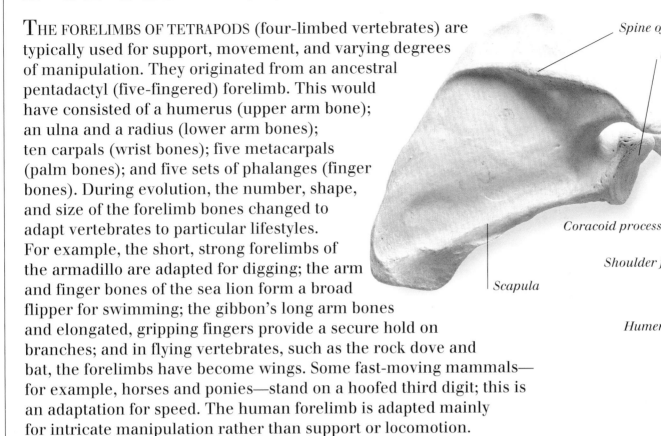

Spine of scapula
Glenoid cavity
Acromion
Head of humerus
Coracoid process
Shoulder joint
Scapula
Humerus
Deltoid tuberosity

ARMADILLO FORELIMB

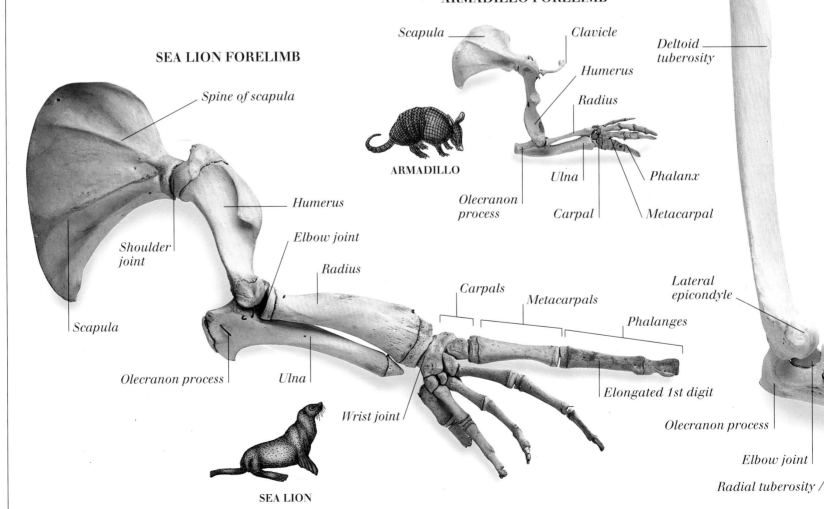

Scapula
Clavicle
Humerus
Radius
ARMADILLO
Ulna
Phalanx
Olecranon process
Carpal
Metacarpal

SEA LION FORELIMB

Spine of scapula
Humerus
Shoulder joint
Elbow joint
Radius
Scapula
Olecranon process
Ulna
Wrist joint
Carpals
Metacarpals
Phalanges
Elongated 1st digit
Lateral epicondyle
Olecranon process
Elbow joint
Radial tuberosity

SEA LION

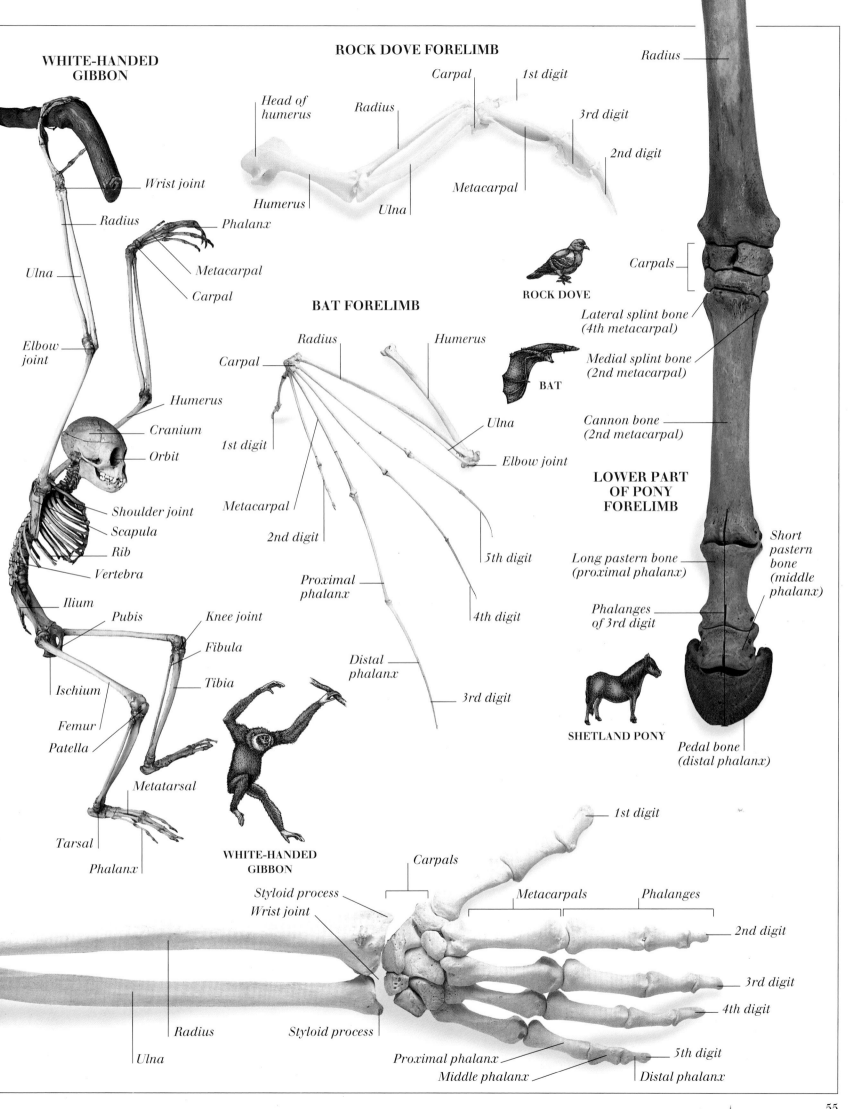

WHITE-HANDED GIBBON

Wrist joint
Radius
Ulna
Elbow joint
Phalanx
Metacarpal
Carpal
Humerus
Cranium
Orbit
Shoulder joint
Scapula
Rib
Vertebra
Ilium
Pubis
Knee joint
Fibula
Ischium
Tibia
Femur
Patella
Metatarsal
Tarsal
Phalanx

WHITE-HANDED GIBBON

ROCK DOVE FORELIMB

Carpal
1st digit
Head of humerus
Radius
3rd digit
2nd digit
Metacarpal
Humerus
Ulna

ROCK DOVE

BAT FORELIMB

Radius
Humerus
Carpal
1st digit
Ulna
Metacarpal
Elbow joint
2nd digit
5th digit
Proximal phalanx
4th digit
Distal phalanx
3rd digit

BAT

Radius

Carpals

Lateral splint bone (4th metacarpal)
Medial splint bone (2nd metacarpal)

Cannon bone (2nd metacarpal)

LOWER PART OF PONY FORELIMB

Long pastern bone (proximal phalanx)
Short pastern bone (middle phalanx)
Phalanges of 3rd digit
Pedal bone (distal phalanx)

SHETLAND PONY

1st digit
Carpals
Styloid process
Wrist joint
Metacarpals
Phalanges
2nd digit
3rd digit
4th digit
Radius
Styloid process
5th digit
Ulna
Proximal phalanx
Middle phalanx
Distal phalanx

Hind limbs

THE HIND LIMBS OF TETRAPODS (four-limbed vertebrates) are more powerful than the forelimbs, and generally provide most of the locomotive force. A typical hind limb consists of a femur (upper leg bone), a tibia and fibula (lower leg bones), tarsals (ankle bones), metatarsals (middle foot bones bones), and phalanges (toe bones). This arrangement, like that of tetrapod forelimbs, evolved from an ancestral pentadactyl (five-fingered) limb, and is adapted to fit particular lifestyles. The seal's short hind limb and elongated foot form a flipper that propels the animal through the water. Long leg and foot bones adapt the serval for pouncing, and the wallaby for balance and a powerful hopping action. The owl's strong hind limbs can be extended to seize prey, and the gibbon uses its long toes to grip branches. The hind limb of the ox has two hoof-tipped toes and fused metatarsals to give strength. The human leg is adapted for an upright posture: the leg bones are long and strong to support body weight, and the long, broad foot provides stability.

HUMAN HIND LIMB

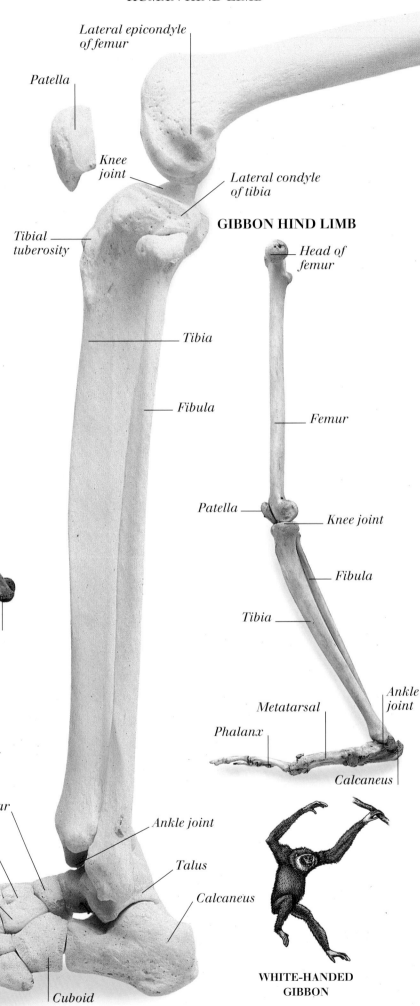

Lateral epicondyle of femur

Patella

Knee joint

Lateral condyle of tibia

Tibial tuberosity

Tibia

Fibula

Ankle joint

Talus

Calcaneus

Navicular

Intermediate cuneiform

Lateral cuneiform

Metatarsal

Digit

Phalanx

Cuboid

GIBBON HIND LIMB

Head of femur

Femur

Patella

Knee joint

Fibula

Tibia

Metatarsal

Phalanx

Ankle joint

Calcaneus

WHITE-HANDED GIBBON

SEAL HIND LIMB

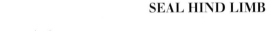

SEAL

Femur

Tibia

Head of femur

Fibula

Tarsals

Metatarsals

Phalanges

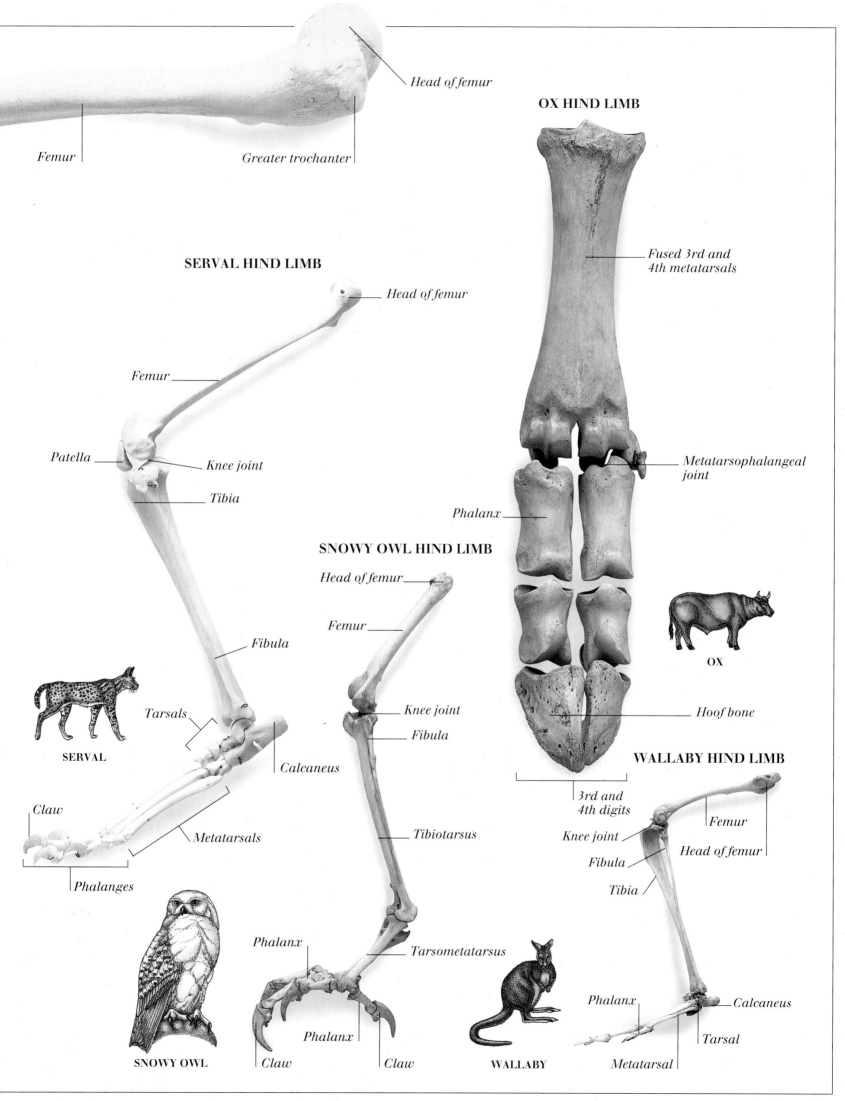

Femur

Head of femur

Greater trochanter

OX HIND LIMB

Fused 3rd and
4th metatarsals

SERVAL HIND LIMB

Head of femur

Femur

Patella

Knee joint

Tibia

Metatarsophalangeal
joint

Phalanx

Fibula

SNOWY OWL HIND LIMB

Head of femur

Femur

Tarsals

SERVAL

Knee joint

Fibula

OX

Calcaneus

Claw

Hoof bone

Metatarsals

WALLABY HIND LIMB

3rd and
4th digits

Knee joint

Femur

Phalanges

Tibiotarsus

Head of femur

Fibula

Tibia

Phalanx

Tarsometatarsus

Phalanx

Calcaneus

Claw

Phalanx

Claw

WALLABY

Metatarsal

Tarsal

SNOWY OWL

Hands and feet

THE HANDS AND FEET of most tetrapods (four-limbed vertebrates) are used for support and movement. However, the human hand is adapted for precise manipulation and grip. The skeleton of the human hand consists of phalanges (finger bones), metacarpals (palm bones), and carpals (wrist bones). The first metacarpal and trapezium bones form a highly mobile saddle joint that gives the thumb its maneuverability. The human foot acts as a lever to propel the body forward, aids balance, and provides support. It consists of 26 bones: seven tarsals (ankle bones), five metatarsals (middle foot bones), and fourteen phalanges (toe bones). The hands and feet of other tetrapods are adapted to their particular lifestyles: the aye-aye's long fingers and toes grip the branches of trees; the penguin's wide foot provides balance and stability on land; and the zebra's leg rests on its third finger, increasing agility and length of stride.

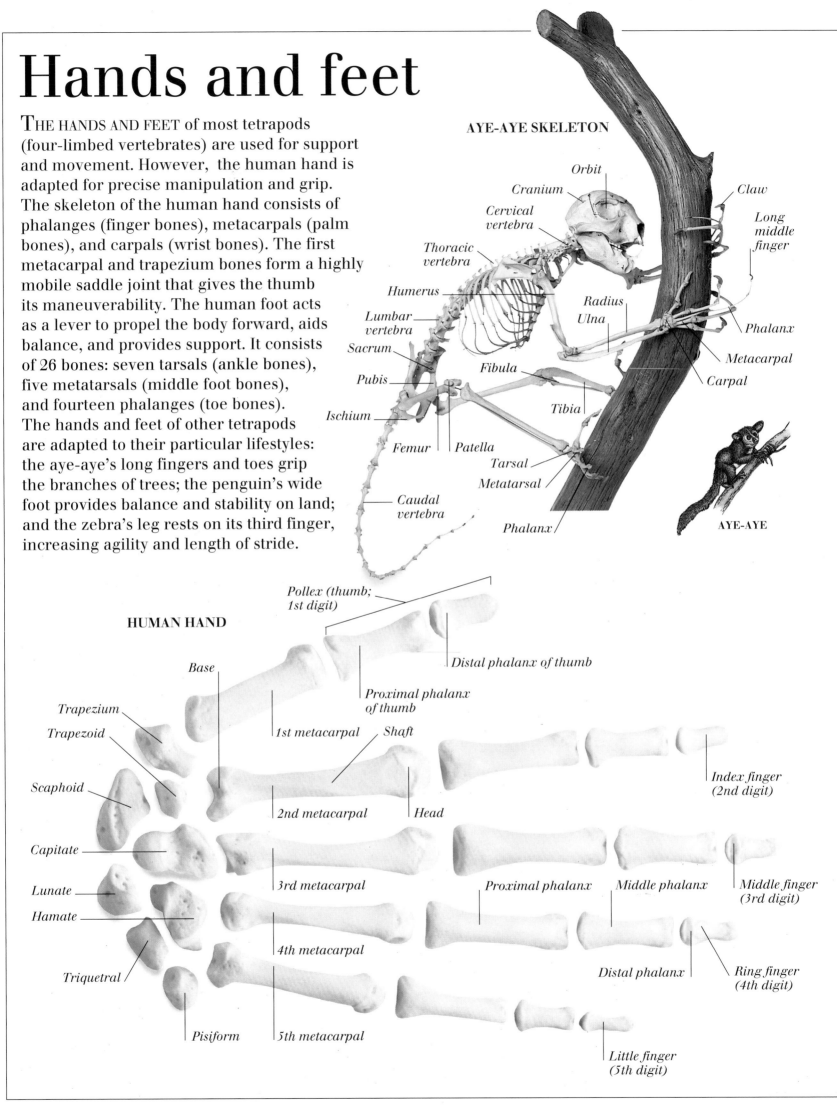

AYE-AYE SKELETON

Orbit
Cranium
Cervical vertebra
Claw
Long middle finger
Thoracic vertebra
Humerus
Radius
Ulna
Lumbar vertebra
Sacrum
Phalanx
Pubis
Fibula
Metacarpal
Carpal
Ischium
Tibia
Femur
Patella
Tarsal
Metatarsal
Caudal vertebra
Phalanx

AYE-AYE

HUMAN HAND

Pollex (thumb; 1st digit)
Distal phalanx of thumb
Base
Proximal phalanx of thumb
Trapezium
Trapezoid
1st metacarpal
Shaft
Index finger (2nd digit)
Scaphoid
2nd metacarpal
Head
Capitate
3rd metacarpal
Proximal phalanx
Middle phalanx
Middle finger (3rd digit)
Lunate
Hamate
4th metacarpal
Distal phalanx
Ring finger (4th digit)
Triquetral
Pisiform
5th metacarpal
Little finger (5th digit)

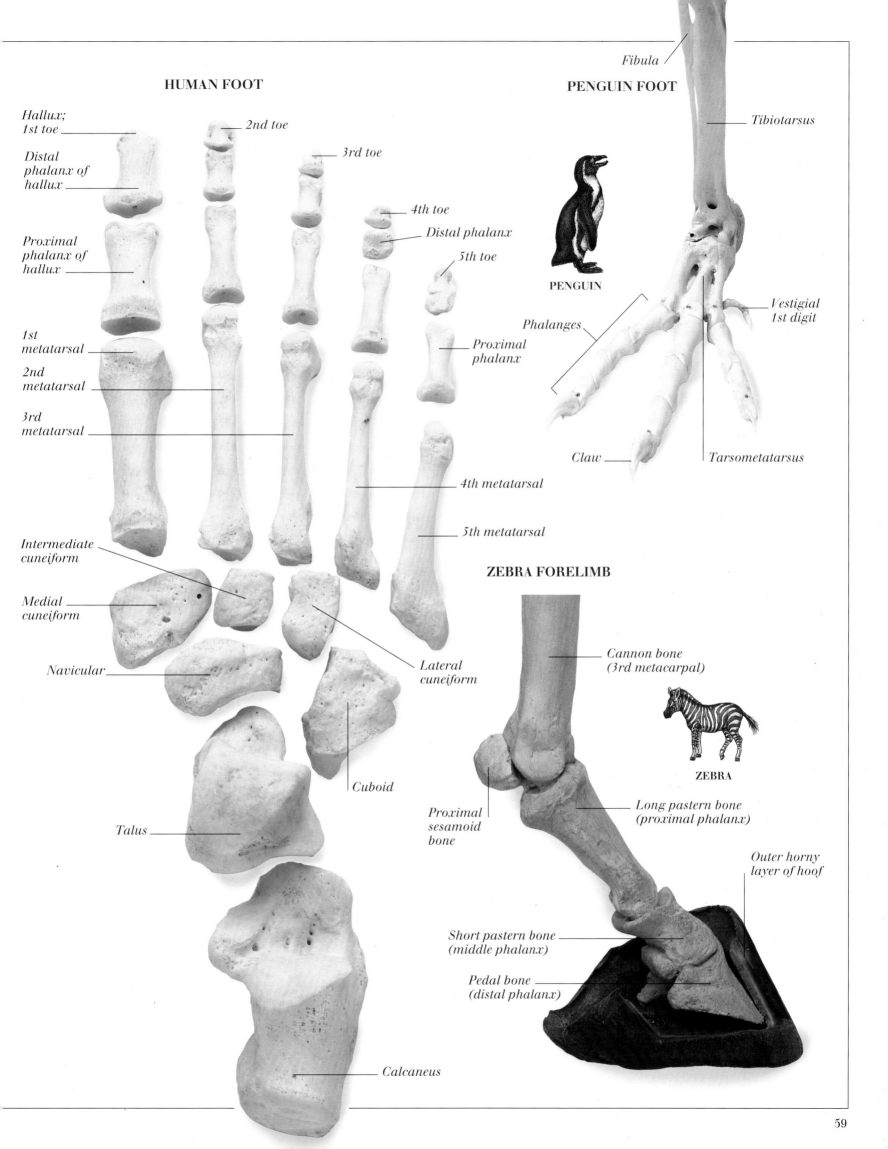

HUMAN FOOT

Hallux;
1st toe

Distal
phalanx of
hallux

2nd toe

3rd toe

Proximal
phalanx of
hallux

4th toe

Distal phalanx

5th toe

1st
metatarsal

2nd
metatarsal

3rd
metatarsal

Proximal
phalanx

4th metatarsal

5th metatarsal

Intermediate
cuneiform

Medial
cuneiform

Navicular

Lateral
cuneiform

Cuboid

Talus

Calcaneus

PENGUIN FOOT

Fibula

Tibiotarsus

PENGUIN

Phalanges

Vestigial
1st digit

Proximal
phalanx

Claw

Tarsometatarsus

ZEBRA FORELIMB

Cannon bone
(3rd metacarpal)

ZEBRA

Long pastern bone
(proximal phalanx)

Proximal
sesamoid
bone

Outer horny
layer of hoof

Short pastern bone
(middle phalanx)

Pedal bone
(distal phalanx)

Index

Acknowledgments

Dorling Kindersley would like to thank:
Dr. Chris Stringer, Dr. Louise Humphrey, and Dr. Peter Andrews at the Department of Paleontology, The Natural History Museum, London; Dr. Gary Sawyer and Dr. Allison Andors of the American Museum of Natural History, New York; Martin Berry, Professor of Anatomy at Guy's Hospital, London for the loan of the human skeleton and the male and female pelvises; George Bridgeman at UMDS for permission to photograph the human skeleton and the male and female pelvises, pp12-15, 52-53; Brandon Broll at the Science Photo Library for editorial help and advice; Edward Bunting and Mary Lindsay for editorial help; Maureen Donovan for advice on labeling the bone marrow micrograph; Stephen Eeley, Jane Pickering, and the staff

of the Oxford University Museum for permission to photograph exhibits; Donald Farr at King's College, London, for editorial help and advice on pelvises; Darren Hill and Mark Wilde for additional design assistance.

Picture credits:

t top; *c* center; *b* bottom; *l* left; *r* right.
The Publisher would like to thank the following for their kind permission to reproduce their photographs: Microscopix/ Andrew Syred 9cl, 16tr, 18tl, 40bl; Science Photo Library/ Scott Camazine 10bl,15t;/ Eric Grave 41b;/ Prof. P. Motta, Department of Anatomy, University La Sapienza, Rome front cover c,15bl,br, 40tr,cr, 41tl;/ David Scharf 41(tr)

Museum credits:
Dorling Kindersley would like to thank: The Natural History Museum, London; The University Museum, Oxford; The Royal Masonic Hospital, London; The University Museum of Zoology, Cambridge; Royal Scottish Museum, Edinburgh; Naturmuseum Senckenburg, Frankfurt.

Dorling Kindersley photographers:
Andy Crawford, Steve Gorton, Sarah Ashun

Makers or owners of models shown in this book: John Dunlop, prepared skeletons: Dogfish skeleton pp 22-23; Salamander skeleton pp 24-25; Monitor Lizard skeleton pp 28-29; Penguin skeleton p 31; Penguin foot p 59

 Somso Modelle, Coburg, Germany: section through buttercup root p 16; section through young woody stem p 17; model of skeleton p 21; hip joint with ligaments/anatomy of hip joint p 42

Additional illustrator: Elizabeth Gray (principal illustrators are credited separately on p 4)

Index: Kay Wright